THE GLUCOSE BREAKTHROUGH

Blood Sugar Balance Has the Power to Change Your Life

By

Harry D. Davis

Copyright © 2023 By Harry D. Davis

This book is a work of nonfiction. While every effort has been made to ensure the accuracy of the information contained herein, the author and publisher assume no responsibility for errors or omissions, or for damages resulting from the use of the information contained herein.

Table of contents

Introduction

Alice was a scientist dedicated to exploring the effects of glucose on the human body. For years, she had been researching and experimenting with different methods of controlling blood sugar levels in people with diabetes.

One day, she made a breakthrough discovery. After many long hours in the lab, she stumbled upon a chemical that had the capacity to regulate blood sugar levels more successfully than any other medication available.

Excited by her findings, Alice couldn't wait to share her discovery with the world. She was aware that the lives of millions of people with diabetes could be changed by this discovery.

But the lab where Alice worked was broken into before she could report her results. Her research notes and the substance she had discovered were taken by the burglar.

Alice felt defeated and was unsure of what to do. She had invested so much time and effort into her research, and now it appeared as though her hard work was all for nothing.

However, a few weeks later, Alice received an anonymous letter. It was from the thief who had stolen her research notes. After expressing regret for their behavior, they gave Alice the compound back.

Once she had control of the compound again, Alice was free to carry on with her studies and finally share her discovery with the world. The discovery of glucose was heralded as one of the most important medical breakthroughs of the decade, and Alice was honored for her commitment and tenacity in the face of difficulty.

An interesting advancement in the field of health and wellbeing is The Glucose Breakthrough. There has been a growing interest in developing new strategies to control this essential molecule as glucose's function in the body has come under more and more scrutiny. The body uses glucose as its main energy source and it is essential for controlling blood sugar levels. However, unbalanced glucose levels can result in a number of health problems, including as diabetes, obesity, and heart disease. By offering creative ways to control glucose levels and advance general health and wellness, The Glucose Breakthrough seeks to solve these issues. In this article, we'll examine the science underlying the "glucose breakthrough" and how it might support people in managing their blood sugar optimally for greater health.

The Glucose Breakthrough's emphasis on individualized methods to glucose management is one of its main features. There is no universal method for controlling glucose levels because every person's body reacts to glucose differently. The Glucose Breakthrough provides a variety of tools and techniques that can be tailored to each person's specific requirements. This entails dietary adjustments, workout regimens, and lifestyle adjustments that are customized to support each person's achievement of ideal glucose levels.

The Glucose Breakthrough uses cutting-edge technology to track and monitor glucose levels, which is another fascinating component of the program. This includes wearable technology that can continuously track blood sugar levels and give feedback on dietary and exercise decisions in real-time. Additionally, developments in machine learning and artificial intelligence are being utilized to evaluate vast amounts of data and offer individualized recommendations for controlling blood sugar levels.

In terms of health and fitness, the Glucose Breakthrough marks a huge advancement. People can take charge of their health and improve results by receiving individualized glycemic management solutions and using technology to detect and monitor glucose levels. We will cover some of the tools and tactics that are available to assist people manage their glucose levels in the parts that follow as well as go into more detail about the science underlying the Glucose Breakthrough.

Chapter 1

Historical Background of Glucose Research

An crucial source of energy for the human body is glucose, a simple sugar. Its study has a long and fascinating history, and it is one of the most fundamental molecules in biology. When people first started learning about the characteristics of plants and their therapeutic uses in antiquity, glucose research had its beginnings.

Ancient Egyptians utilized honey as a sweetener for food and beverages and were the first to record its sweetening abilities. They were also aware of the healing properties of honey in the treatment of wounds and other illnesses. But glucose was initially recognized as a separate chemical by the Greeks. The phrase "glukus," which the Greek physician Dioscorides described as a sweet, white fluid taken from figs, is thought to be the ancestor of the modern word "glucose."

The use of sugar as a sweetener increased during the Middle Ages, as did the study of plants and their qualities. Arab researchers made important advances in the study of sugar, creating fresh techniques for removing sugar from sugarcane and purifying it into white sugar crystals.

Discovery glucose in the blood

With the discovery of glucose in human blood in the late 18th and early 19th centuries, the modern research of glucose got underway. Antoine Lavoisier, a French surgeon, discovered in 1780 that animal blood contained a component that, when heated with sulfuric acid, could be transformed into carbon dioxide and water. He referred to it as "respirable gas" before identifying it as glucose.

Lavoisier's findings were corroborated by English physician Matthew Dobson in 1801, who found that human blood likewise contained glucose. However, the significance of glucose in the human body was not fully understood until the middle of the 19th century.

The German physician Claude Bernard discovered gluconeogenesis, or the production of glucose by the liver from non-carbohydrate sources, in 1855. This was a major finding since it showed that the body could manufacture glucose on its own and not merely as a byproduct of digestion.

Discovery of insulin

In addition to revolutionizing the management of diabetes, the 1921 discovery of insulin increased our knowledge of glucose metabolism. Before the discovery of insulin, diabetes was a fatal condition with no reliable cure. Injecting a pancreas extract into diabetic dogs could lower their blood glucose levels, as discovered in 1921 by Canadian doctors Frederick Banting and Charles Best. Later studies revealed that this extract, which they dubbed insulin, was efficient in treating diabetes in people.

Significant strides in the understanding of glucose metabolism and the management of diabetes were made after the discovery of insulin. It also sparked the creation of fresh techniques for determining blood glucose levels, including the still-in-use glucose tolerance test.

Role Of Glucose In Generating Energy

We have learned a lot about how glucose functions in the creation of energy thanks to the 20th century's continuing study of glucose metabolism. The citric acid cycle, commonly referred to as the Krebs cycle, is a sequence of chemical reactions that generate energy from glucose and other molecules. It was first discovered in the 1930s by the German biochemist Hans Krebs.

Melvin Calvin, an American biochemist, and his colleagues explored photosynthesis in the 1950s and 1960s. Photosynthesis is the biological process in which plants use sunlight as a source of energy to convert carbon dioxide and water into glucose.The Calvin cycle, a chain of chemical events that causes plants to create glucose, was discovered as a result of their research.

Advances In The Study Of Glucose

Through the 20th and into the 21st centuries, research on glucose continued to advance. The 1970s saw ground-breaking studies on how dietary carbohydrates affect cholesterol levels and heart disease undertaken by American scientist David Kritchevsky and his associates. A high-carbohydrate diet has been linked to higher levels of low-density lipoprotein (LDL), a kind of cholesterol that is a risk factor for heart disease, according to their research.

Researchers started looking at how glucose affected the onset of diabetes and other metabolic problems in the 1980s and 1990s. As a result of this research, the condition known as insulin resistance, which causes the body's cells to become less receptive to insulin and may ultimately result in diabetes, was identified.

Our understanding of glucose metabolism has greatly improved over the past few years as a result of developments in genetics and molecular biology. Researchers have discovered novel molecular pathways that control the body's glucose levels as well as multiple genes that are involved in glucose regulation and metabolism.

The research of glucose is now being done in other creatures as well as the environment, going beyond just human physiology. For instance, studies are being conducted on the function of glucose in microbial communities, as well as its utilization in biofuels and other commercial processes.

Glucose research has a long and fascinating history that dates back to antiquity. Researchers have contributed much to our knowledge of glucose metabolism and its function in human health and disease over the years. The discovery of insulin in 1921 transformed diabetes care, and important strides in our understanding of glucose regulation and metabolism have been made as a result of developments in genetics and molecular biology.

Researchers are constantly looking for innovative ways to better understand how glucose affects human health and disease in the subject of glucose research today. It is expected that the study of glucose will continue to be a busy research and discovery topic for many years to come thanks to ongoing technological advancements and new instruments for researching glucose at the molecular level.

Why Is The Glucose Breakthrough Important?

Our body's main source of energy is a form of sugar called glucose. It is necessary for several body processes, including cell proliferation, muscular contraction, and brain function. Therefore, a development in the regulation and metabolism of glucose could have a big impact on people's health and happiness. We shall talk about the significance of the glucose breakthrough and how it affects our life in this book.

1.Better Understanding of Glucose Metabolism Mechanisms:
Improving our understanding of glucose metabolism mechanisms is one of the most significant benefits

of the glucose breakthrough. The process through which our body breaks down glucose and transforms it into energy is referred to as glucose metabolism. The more we comprehend this process, the more we may create interventions to improve it and prevent or treat disorders like diabetes and metabolic syndrome that are linked to glucose metabolism.

2. Creating New Diabetes Treatments:

Diabetes, a metabolic condition that affects millions of people globally, is a priority right now. It happens when the body is unable to adequately use or create insulin, a hormone that aids in controlling blood glucose levels. By identifying novel pharmacological targets or expanding our knowledge of how current medicines function, a glucose breakthrough can aid in the creation of new diabetic medications.

3. Increasing athletic performance:

During activity, glucose is a vital source of energy for muscles. Therefore, a development in glucose metabolism may have important effects on how well athletes perform. Athletes can optimize their training and diet routines to improve performance by being aware of how the body uses glucose while exercising.

4. Improved Management of Metabolic Disorders:

Diabetes and metabolic syndrome are two of the most prevalent and expensive health issues in the world. By enhancing our comprehension of the underlying mechanisms underlying these ailments, locating novel therapeutic choices, and creating more potent preventive measures, a glucose breakthrough can assist us in managing them more effectively.

5. Improving Brain Function:

Since glucose is the brain's main energy source, proper glucose metabolism is essential for brain health. A glucose discovery could increase our understanding of how the brain uses glucose and pave the way for the creation of novel treatments or preventions for neurodegenerative conditions like Alzheimer's disease.

6. Preventing Chronic Diseases:

The regulation of glucose metabolism has a key role in the development of chronic conditions such cancer, obesity, and cardiovascular disease. The processes by which glucose metabolism contributes to the emergence of various disorders can be determined with the aid of a glucose breakthrough. As a result, we may be able to create more successful preventative and treatment plans for certain chronic illnesses.

7. Personalized Nutrition and Medicine:

A glucose breakthrough may likewise have significant effects on these fields. Healthcare practitioners can modify treatment regimens and dietary suggestions to improve patient outcomes by better knowing how a patient's body metabolizes glucose. This individualized strategy may result in more efficient and effective medical interventions, lowering the possibility of negative side effects and enhancing patient quality of life.

8. Lowering Healthcare expenditures:

Diabetes and other metabolic illnesses come with significant and rising healthcare expenditures. In order to lessen the toll that these diseases take on people and healthcare systems, we may build prevention and treatment plans that are more successful thanks to a glucose breakthrough. We can lower healthcare expenditures and enhance patient outcomes by preventing and controlling metabolic diseases.

9. Promoting Better Public Health:

A glucose breakthrough can support better public health by increasing our understanding of glucose metabolism and its function in human health. Implementing public health initiatives to lower the prevalence of metabolic diseases, such as encouraging good food and exercise, and raising knowledge of the significance of glucose metabolism for general health are a few examples of what this could include.

10. research and Technology Advancement:

Finally, a glucose discovery could contribute to the overall advancement of research and technology. The creation of novel instruments and methods for investigating glucose metabolism may result in fresh understandings in domains including molecular biology, biochemistry, and physiology. New technologies and treatments for a variety of illnesses and disorders might result from this.

The glucose breakthrough is significant for a number of reasons, including enhancing our comprehension of glucose metabolism, creating novel therapies for metabolic disorders, enhancing brain function, enhancing athletic performance, preventing chronic diseases, promoting personalized nutrition and medicine, lowering healthcare costs, enhancing public health, and advancing science and technology. Therefore, continuing this type of study is crucial to enhancing human health and wellbeing.

Chapter 2

Understanding Glucose

A simple molecule called glucose, commonly referred to as a monosaccharide, is essential to human metabolism. It is the body's main source of energy and a significant part of many foods, including grains, fruits, and vegetables. This article will examine the fundamental characteristics of glucose, its function in human physiology, and the different elements that might affect the body's glucose levels.

Specifications of Glucose

The chemical formula of glucose, which is a sugar consisting of six carbon atoms, is $C_6H_{12}O_6$.. It is categorized as an aldohexose because it has six carbon atoms and an aldehyde functional group. The molecular weight of glucose is 180.16 g/mol, and its density is 1.54 g/cm3. It is a white, crystalline substance with considerable water solubility and only moderate solubility in ethanol.

Glucose is a dextro-rotatory enantiomer, which means that when polarized light is focused on it, it rotates to the right. It gets its name "dextrose" from this. The second form of glucose, which rotates light to the left, is also present in nature as a mixture of two enantiomers. The majority of foods and the human body include a mixture known as "glucose" in this form.

In Human Physiology, Glucose

Glucose is a key component of human physiology because it is the body's cells' main source of energy. When we eat carbs, our bodies convert them into glucose molecules, which are then taken into the bloodstream. This causes the pancreas to release insulin, allowing the glucose to enter the cells and be used as energy.

The body can utilize glucose in a variety of ways. It can be converted into the molecule that powers the majority of cellular functions, ATP (adenosine triphosphate), by oxidation. It can also be utilized to create glycogen, which is predominantly kept in the liver and muscles and is the body's type of glucose storage. When the body needs energy, such as during activity or times of starvation, glycogen can be converted into glucose.

Glucose serves as an energy source in addition to participating in a number of other physiological functions. It is a part of numerous complex carbohydrates, such as starch and cellulose, which make up the majority of the dietary fiber in our bodies. A number of significant compounds, such as glycoproteins (proteins with linked carbohydrate molecules) and nucleic acids (DNA and RNA), are also synthesized using glucose.

Control of Blood Glucose

To guarantee that cells always have an energy supply, the body closely controls glucose levels. After a meal, when blood sugar levels rise, insulin is released to encourage glucose uptake into cells and encourage the storage of extra glucose as glycogen. Glucagon is released to encourage the breakdown of glycogen and the release of glucose into the bloodstream when blood glucose levels fall during fasting or exercise.

But when the body's control over glucose levels is thrown off, issues may result. For instance, in those who have diabetes, the body is unable to adequately make or react to insulin, which results in elevated blood sugar levels (hyperglycemia). This has the potential to harm organs, nerves, and blood vessels over time, among other health issues.

The body's glucose levels can also be impacted by a number of other variables. For instance, stress and illness can temporarily raise blood sugar levels because these conditions induce the body to generate stress hormones, which in turn trigger the liver to release glucose into the bloodstream. The blood glucose levels of various drugs, including some diuretics and corticosteroids, can also rise.

Checking Blood Glucose Levels
Monitoring blood glucose levels is a crucial element of managing diabetes for those who have it. A blood glucose meter can be used to quantify the amount of glucose in a little drop of blood taken from a finger prick. There are also devices for continuous glucose monitoring (CGM) that use a tiny sensor implanted

under the skin to continuously monitor glucose levels throughout the day.

It is less frequent for those without diabetes to check their blood glucose levels. For those who have certain risk factors, such as a family history of diabetes, obesity, or a sedentary lifestyle, it might be advised. Two frequent tests used to check for diabetes and other conditions related to glucose are oral glucose tolerance tests and fasting blood glucose tests.

As the body's main source of energy, glucose is an essential component of human physiology. The body closely controls it to guarantee a steady flow of energy, and a breakdown in this control can result in a number of health issues. For diabetics and those at risk of developing illnesses connected to high blood sugar, monitoring glucose levels is crucial.

What Is Glucose

A necessary chemical that is crucial to the functioning of the human body is glucose. It is a simple sugar that gives cells energy and serves as the main source of fuel for the organs, including the brain. Given that it is delivered to cells all over the body by the bloodstream, glucose is also known as blood sugar. Glucose will be covered in this article along with its definition, production process, uses, and significance for preserving health.

Define glucose.

A monosaccharide, or simple sugar made up of only one sugar molecule, is glucose. Given that it has six carbon atoms, twelve hydrogen atoms, and six oxygen atoms, it is also categorized as a hexose. The most prevalent and necessary carbohydrate in the human body, glucose is used by cells as an energy source.

Plants produce glucose during photosynthesis, which serves as their main source of energy. When plants are consumed by animals, their digestive systems break down the glucose, which is then taken into the circulation and sent to the cells' energy-producing organs. When glucose intake is minimal, glucose is also generated in the liver and delivered into the bloodstream to maintain blood sugar levels.

Exactly how is glucose made?

During photosynthesis, when carbon dioxide and water are transformed into glucose and oxygen with the aid of sunlight, plants make glucose. In the chloroplasts of plant cells, the process of photosynthesis takes place. Chlorophyll receives light energy and uses it to change carbon dioxide and water into glucose and oxygen.

In mammals, the breakdown of carbohydrates like starch and glycogen results in the production of glucose. When we consume carbs, our digestive system converts them into simple sugars like glucose, which are then taken into the circulation and sent to the cells for energy. The process of glycogenolysis, in which glycogen is broken down into glucose, also produces glucose in the liver.

The uses of glucose

Providing energy to cells is glucose's main purpose. The liver, heart, and muscles, as well as the brain and other organs, mostly rely on it for energy. Through a process known as cellular respiration, glucose is taken up by cells all over the body and transformed into energy. This process is carried out by the bloodstream.

In addition to giving off energy, glucose aids in the body's creation of other critical chemicals. For instance, glycogen is created from glucose and is stored in the liver and muscles where it serves as a backup energy source. The components of DNA and RNA, known as nucleotides, are also produced using glucose.

The significance of glucose in preserving health

For optimal health, blood glucose levels must be kept normal. A sophisticated mechanism comprising hormones like insulin and glucagon helps the body control blood glucose levels.

The pancreas secretes the hormone insulin, which instructs cells to take up glucose from the bloodstream and control blood sugar levels. When blood sugar levels are high, the hormone insulin is released into the bloodstream, signaling cells to take up glucose and lowering blood sugar levels.

Another hormone made by the pancreas, glucagon, controls blood glucose levels by telling the liver to release glucose that has been stored in the body. Glucagon is released into the bloodstream in response to low blood glucose levels, telling the liver to release glucose from storage and raising blood glucose levels.

Since both high and low blood glucose levels can have harmful consequences on the body, maintaining normal blood glucose levels is crucial for optimal health. While hypoglycemia, or low blood sugar, can result in symptoms like lightheadedness, confusion, and seizures, hyperglycemia, or high blood sugar, can result in consequences like diabetes.

Diabetes and Glucose

Diabetes is a chronic illness brought on when the body struggles to control blood glucose levels. The two main subcategories of diabetes are type 1 and type 2.

The immune system targets and kills the cells in the pancreas that make insulin in type 1 diabetes, an autoimmune condition. Because of this, people with type 1 diabetes need to inject themselves with insulin or use an insulin pump to control their blood sugar levels.

When the body develops an insulin resistance or is unable to produce enough insulin to maintain healthy blood glucose levels, type 2 diabetes develops. This particular form of diabetes is frequently linked to unhealthy eating habits, inactivity, and obesity.

Diabetes consequences can include damage to the eyes, kidneys, and nerves due to high blood glucose levels. The risk of cardiovascular disease, stroke, and other health issues can all be heightened by diabetes.

In order to treat diabetes, normal blood glucose levels must be maintained through a combination of medication, lifestyle modifications, and routine blood glucose monitoring. This may entail taking insulin or other medications orally that improve how well the body uses insulin, as well as making changes to one's lifestyle through frequent exercise and a nutritious diet.

Exercise and Glucose

The body needs extra energy when exercising, and one of the main fuel sources for the muscles is glucose. Exercise causes the body to release chemicals like adrenaline and cortisol, which tell the liver to release glucose from storage into the bloodstream.

During exercise, the muscles absorb glucose and use cellular respiration to turn it into energy. The body boosts its oxygen intake during exercise to match the increased demand since this mechanism is more effective when oxygen is available.

Regular physical activity has been demonstrated to enhance the body's utilization of glucose and can aid in lowering the risk of type 2 diabetes. Exercise is crucial for managing diabetes since it can assist those with the disease in controlling blood glucose levels.

Diabetes Testing

The amount of glucose in the blood can be measured using a blood glucose meter, which takes a small sample of blood to do so. Diabetes patients frequently use this to routinely check their blood glucose levels.

Self-monitoring of blood glucose (SMBG) and continuous glucose monitoring (CGM) are the two primary categories of blood glucose measurement. While CGM includes wearing a device that continually monitors blood glucose levels throughout the day, SMBG entails measuring blood glucose levels at home using a blood glucose meter.

Glucose levels in urine and saliva can also be assessed in addition to blood tests. These techniques are not frequently used to manage diabetes because they are less accurate than blood glucose measurement.

glucose is a necessary chemical that is crucial to the functioning of the human body. It is a simple sugar that gives cells energy and serves as the main source of fuel for the organs, including the brain. In order to keep blood sugar levels stable, glucose is created by plants during photosynthesis as well as in the liver and delivered into the bloodstream.

Since both high and low blood glucose levels can have harmful consequences on the body, maintaining normal blood glucose levels is crucial for optimal health. Diabetes is a chronic disease that can cause a variety of issues when the body is unable to control blood glucose levels.

A crucial tool for controlling diabetes and preserving good health is glucose testing. People can help prevent the difficulties linked to high blood glucose levels and maintain good health by frequently monitoring their blood glucose levels and changing their lifestyles as necessary.

How Does The Body Metabolize Glucose?

The process through which glucose is digested and converted into energy is known as glucose metabolism. Multiple processes make up this process, which is controlled by a sophisticated network of hormones and enzymes.

The detailed metabolism of glucose, including how it enters cells, how it is converted to energy, and how extra glucose is stored in the body, will be covered in this article. We'll also look at how hormones like glucagon and insulin control how our bodies use glucose.

Transport of Glucose into Cells

Transporting glucose into cells is the initial step in the metabolism of glucose. A family of proteins called glucose transporters, or GLUTs, transfer glucose across cell membranes. There are various distinct GLUT subtypes, but GLUT4 is crucial for glucose metabolism.

Muscle and adipose (fat) tissue are the main sites of GLUT4 expression, which is also in charge of the majority of glucose uptake in these tissues. An important factor in controlling GLUT4 activity is insulin. After a meal, for example, high insulin levels encourage GLUT4 to move from intracellular vesicles to the cell membrane, where it can carry glucose into the cell. This is a crucial process for preserving the body's glucose homeostasis.

Glucose can either be saved for later use or utilised for energy production after it has entered the cell.

Blood Sugar Metabolism

Glycolysis and the citric acid cycle, commonly referred to as the Krebs cycle or the tricarboxylic acid cycle, are the two primary processes for the metabolism of glucose. Let's examine each of these routes in more detail.

Glycolysis

The first step in the metabolism of glucose is called glycolysis, and it takes place in the cell's cytoplasm. The transformation of glucose into pyruvate, a three-carbon molecule, takes place over the course of ten enzyme processes. A little quantity of ATP (adenosine triphosphate), the main form of energy used by cells, is produced during glycolysis.

The energy investment phase and the energy payback phase are two segments that make up the 10 steps of glycolysis. Two molecules of ATP are used in the energy investment phase to activate glucose, which is subsequently broken down into two molecules of glyceraldehyde 3-phosphate. These molecules are turned into pyruvate during the energy payout phase, which also results in the production of two molecules of the high-energy electron transporter NADH and four molecules of ATP.

The following diagram illustrates how glycolysis functions as a whole:

Pyruvate + 2 NADH + 2 ATP + 2 H+ = glucose + 2 NAD+ + 2 ADP + 2 Pi.

Later steps of the metabolism of glucose can employ the NADH produced by glycolysis to produce more ATP.

The Cycle of Citric Acid

The citric acid cycle, which takes place in the cell's mitochondria, is the second stage of glucose metabolism. Pyruvate dehydrogenase uses the pyruvate produced during glycolysis to enter the mitochondria and transform it into acetyl-CoA. After entering the citric acid cycle, which is a chain of eight enzymatic processes, acetyl-CoA is converted to carbon dioxide (CO_2) and NADH and FADH2 (flavin adenine dinucleotide), which serve as high-energy electron carriers, are produced.

The following diagram illustrates how the citric acid cycle reacts as a whole:

Acetyl-CoA: 2 CO2 + 3 NADH + FADH2 + GTP + CoA-SH 3 NAD+ + FAD + GDP + Pi

The oxidative phosphorylation procedure, which we will go over in more detail later, uses the NADH and FADH2 produced by the citric acid cycle to create ATP.

The Control of the Metabolism of Glucose

A sophisticated network of hormones and enzymes carefully controls glucose metabolism. Insulin and glucagon are the two primary hormones involved in the metabolism of glucose.

The pancreatic beta cells release insulin in response to high blood glucose levels, such as those that occur after a meal. Insulin stimulates GLUT4 translocation to the cell membrane, promoting glucose absorption into cells. By promoting glycogen synthesis, it also encourages glucose storage in the liver and muscle tissue.

On the other hand, glucagon is created by the pancreatic alpha cells in reaction to low blood sugar, such as during fasting or exercise. In order to release glucose into the bloodstream, glucagon induces the breakdown of glycogen in the liver. Additionally, it promotes gluconeogenesis, the process of producing glucose from non-carbohydrate sources like amino acids and fatty acids.

AMP-activated protein kinase (AMPK) is a key regulator of glucose metabolism. When cellular energy levels are low, as they are during exercise or fasting, AMPK is triggered, which increases the uptake and utilisation of glucose in muscle tissue. Additionally, it encourages fatty acid oxidation and reduces the liver's ability to produce glucose.

Phosphofructokinase-1 (PFK-1), an essential enzyme in the metabolism of glucose, catalyzes the third phase of glycolysis. PFK-1 is blocked by ATP, which denotes a high level of cellular energy, and activated by AMP, which denotes a low level of cellular energy. This makes it easier to guarantee that glycolysis only kicks in when energy is required.

Metabolism of Glycogen

Glycogen, a branching polymer of glucose molecules, is a form of storage for extra glucose in the body. When energy is required, glycogen can be quickly broken down to produce glucose. The liver and muscle tissue are the primary sites where glycogen is predominantly stored.

In reaction to elevated insulin levels, glycogen synthesis takes place in the liver and muscle tissue. The enzyme glycogen synthase transforms glucose into glucose-6-phosphate, which is ultimately transformed into glycogen.

Low blood glucose levels and the hormone glucagon both promote glycogenolysis, or the breakdown of glycogen. Glucose-6-phosphate is created in the liver when glycogen is broken down, and it is subsequently transformed into glucose and delivered into the bloodstream. Glycogen is converted in muscle tissue into glucose-6-phosphate, which is required to power muscular contraction.

Phosphorylation by Oxidation

Oxidative phosphorylation, which takes place in the cell's mitochondria, is the last step in the metabolism of glucose. In order to complete this process, electrons must be transferred from NADH and FADH2 to a chain of electron carriers called the electron transport chain. A proton gradient is produced by pumping protons across the inner mitochondrial membrane using the energy released during the transport of electrons. After passing through ATP synthase, the protons return across the membrane and produce ATP.

Oxidative phosphorylation can be seen as the following:

$$NAD+ + H2O + ATP = NADH + H+ + 1/2\ O2 + ADP + Pi$$

ATP synthase activity and the number of protons pumped across the membrane determine how many ATP molecules are produced by oxidative phosphorylation. In general, each NADH and FADH2 molecule produces 2.5 and 1.5 ATP molecules, respectively.

Disorders of the Metabolism of Glucose

When the system of hormones and enzymes that controls glucose metabolism is disturbed, disorders of glucose metabolism can develop. Diabetes mellitus and hypoglycemia are two frequently occurring diseases of glucose metabolism.

The body's ability to appropriately manage blood glucose levels is impaired in diabetes mellitus. There are two fundamental types of diabetes: type 1 and type 2.

A lack of insulin production results from the pancreas' beta cells being damaged in type 1 diabetes, an autoimmune condition. High blood glucose levels are the outcome, and over time, they can harm the body. Both insulin injections and an insulin pump are used to treat type 1 diabetes.

High blood glucose levels result from type 2 diabetes, which is a condition in which the body grows resistant to insulin. It can be controlled with lifestyle modifications and medicine, and it is frequently linked to obesity and a sedentary lifestyle.

An abnormally low blood glucose level is referred to as hypoglycemia. Numerous things, such as an excessive amount of insulin, a protracted fast, and specific drugs, can contribute to it. Hypoglycemia can cause seizures, disorientation, and lightheadedness. Consuming glucose-containing meals and beverages, such as fruit juice, glucose tablets, or candies, is part of the treatment process. Glucagon injections may be necessary in more serious situations to elevate blood glucose levels.

A number of enzymes and metabolic pathways work together to convert glucose into energy in the process known as glucose metabolism. An intricate network of hormones and enzymes closely controls the process to make sure that energy is supplied when it is required and stored when it is not.

When the system of hormones and enzymes that controls glucose metabolism is disturbed, conditions including diabetes mellitus and hypoglycemia can develop. These problems need to be managed carefully since they can have catastrophic repercussions.

Understanding glucose metabolism is crucial for developing new treatments for a variety of metabolic diseases as well as for treating problems of glucose metabolism. To increase our knowledge of the fundamental mechanisms of glucose metabolism and create new treatments for metabolic illnesses, it is crucial to do ongoing research in this area.

Insulin's Function in Glucose Regulation

The body uses glucose as its main energy source, and controlling glucose levels is crucial for supporting physiological processes. The pancreas secretes the hormone insulin, which is essential for maintaining glucose homeostasis. By encouraging glucose uptake into cells, encouraging glycogen synthesis, and inhibiting gluconeogenesis, insulin controls blood sugar levels. The function of insulin in controlling blood sugar will be briefly discussed in this essay, along with its modes of action and the physiological mechanisms that support glucose homeostasis.

Synthesis and Secretion of Insulin

The beta cells of the pancreas, which are found in the islets of Langerhans, produce and secrete insulin. In the endoplasmic reticulum, where it is initially created as a preproinsulin molecule, insulin is synthesized. The signal peptide in preproinsulin is then broken down in the Golgi apparatus, where it is converted into proinsulin. After being packaged into secretory vesicles, proinsulin is then further processed by cleaving the C-peptide to produce insulin and a fragment of the C-peptide. As a marker of insulin production, the C-peptide is co-secreted with insulin.

A complicated interplay between glucose, amino acids, and other hormones controls the secretion of insulin. The glucose transporter GLUT2 facilitates glucose absorption by beta cells, which is the key stimulus for insulin release. Once inside the beta cell, glucose is digested through the glycolytic pathway, which raises the levels of ATP inside the beta cell. Calcium influx and membrane depolarization are caused by the activation of ATP-sensitive potassium (KATP) channels by an increase in ATP. Insulin is released into the bloodstream as a result of insulin exocytosis being triggered by calcium influx.

Other foods, such amino acids, can also trigger insulin production in addition to glucose. Specific transporters carry amino acids into beta cells, where their processing results in the production of metabolic intermediates that can increase insulin secretion. Additionally, other hormones such as glucagon-like peptide-1 (GLP-1) induce the release of insulin. In response to meal consumption, intestinal L-cells release GLP-1, which acts on beta cells to boost insulin output.

Pathway for Insulin Receptor Signaling

The insulin receptor, a transmembrane protein that is a member of the tyrosine kinase receptor family, is the mechanism through which insulin acts on target tissues. Two alpha subunits and two beta subunits make up the insulin receptor; they are joined together by disulfide bonds. The insulin-binding domain is found in the alpha subunits, which are found extracellularly, whereas the tyrosine kinase domain is found in the beta subunits, which are found intracellularly.

The beta subunits' tyrosine kinase activity is activated by a conformational shift brought on by insulin binding to the alpha subunits. Tyrosine residues in the beta subunits are subsequently autophosphorylated as a result, producing docking sites for signaling molecules downstream. The phosphatidylinositol 3-kinase (PI3K) pathway is one of the main downstream signaling pathways that the insulin receptor signaling activates.

The regulatory subunit of PI3K binds to phosphorylated tyrosine residues on the insulin receptor, activating the PI3K pathway. As a result, phosphatidylinositol-4,5-bisphosphate (PIP2) is phosphorylated to produce phosphatidylinositol-3,4,5-trisphosphate (PIP3), which is then activated by the catalytic subunit of PI3K. Mechanistic target of rapamycin complex 1 (mTORC1) and protein kinase B (Akt), two downstream signaling molecules, are then activated by PIP3.

The Effects of Insulin on Glucose Metabolism

In addition to encouraging glucose absorption into cells and preventing gluconeogenesis, insulin also controls glucose metabolism by increasing glycogen synthesis.

Glucose Uptake

By increasing the translocation of glucose transporter type 4 (GLUT4) to the plasma membrane, insulin facilitates the absorption of glucose into cells. A crucial step in insulin-mediated glucose absorption is GLUT4's translocation to the plasma membrane, which is largely expressed in adipose tissue, skeletal muscle, and cardiac muscle.

The PI3K pathway controls GLUT4's translocation to the plasma membrane. Akt substrate 160 (AS160), a Rab GTPase-activating protein, is phosphorylated and activated as a result of Akt activation. As GLUT4-containing vesicles are transported to the plasma membrane, AS160 controls the activity of the Rab proteins. The activation of Rab proteins by Akt's phosphorylation of AS160 aids in the translocation of GLUT4 to the plasma membrane.

Gluconeogenesis

Insulin prevents the liver from producing glucose from non-carbohydrate sources, a process known as gluconeogenesis. Gluconeogenesis is a crucial mechanism for keeping blood glucose levels stable during fasting or exercise, however in those with diabetes, excessive gluconeogenesis can lead to hyperglycemia.

Phosphoenolpyruvate carboxykinase (PEPCK) and glucose-6-phosphatase (G6Pase), two essential enzymes involved in gluconeogenesis, are suppressed in insulin's ability to limit gluconeogenesis. Additionally, insulin encourages the liver's uptake of lactate and pyruvate, which can act as substitute substrates for the synthesis of glucose.

Synthesis of Glycogen
Glycogen synthesis, the process by which glucose is transformed into glycogen and stored in the liver and muscle, is facilitated by insulin. When you fast or exercise, glucose stored in your body's glycogen might be released.

By turning on glycogen synthase, the enzyme that catalyzes the conversion of glucose-6-phosphate to glycogen, insulin promotes glycogen production. By preventing glycogen phosphorylase, the enzyme that catalyzes the conversion of glycogen to glucose-6-phosphate, insulin also prevents glycogen degradation.

Insulin Secretion Control

To maintain glucose homeostasis, insulin secretion is strictly controlled. Glucose, amino acids, and other hormones, including as glucagon and incretins, interact intricately to control insulin secretion.

Insulin production is primarily stimulated by glucose, and the incretin effect is a feedback mechanism that controls how much insulin is produced. The term "incretin effect" describes how insulin release is amplified in response to oral glucose as opposed to intravenous glucose. Incretin hormones, such as GLP-1 and glucose-dependent insulinotropic polypeptide (GIP), which are produced by intestinal L-cells in response to food intake, are responsible for mediating this effect.

Increasing intracellular cAMP levels and activating the PI3K pathway are two ways that incretin hormones influence beta cells to promote insulin production. The regulation of glucose homeostasis is further supported by incretin hormones' inhibition of glucagon secretion.

The pancreatic alpha cells secrete the hormone glucagon, which encourages the liver to create glucose through gluconeogenesis and glycogenolysis. Insulin lowers alpha cell activity, inhibits glucagon release, and promotes the transformation of proglucagon into GLP-1 and other bioactive peptides.

Other hormones, including as catecholamines, growth hormone, and cortisol, have an impact on the control of insulin secretion. Depending on the situation and the balance of other signals in the body, these hormones can either promote or block the release of insulin.

The Metabolism Of Glucose And Insulin Is Dysregulated.

Type 1 and type 2 diabetes, metabolic syndrome, and obesity are just a few of the metabolic illnesses that can develop as a result of insulin and glucose metabolism dysregulation.

Insulin shortage results from the pancreatic beta cells being destroyed in type 1 diabetes, an autoimmune condition. Insulin therapy is necessary for type 1 diabetic patients to maintain glucose homeostasis.

Insulin resistance and dysfunctional beta cells are two features of type 2 diabetes, which causes hyperglycemia. Obesity and other metabolic abnormalities are frequently linked to type 2 diabetes, which is a serious global public health concern.

An accumulation of metabolic abnormalities known as the metabolic syndrome include central obesity, insulin resistance, hypertension, dyslipidemia, and hypertension. The metabolic syndrome is linked to higher rates of morbidity and mortality and is a risk factor for type 2 diabetes and cardiovascular disease.

Obesity is linked to persistent low-grade inflammation, dysregulation of adipokines, hormones secreted by adipose tissue that regulate metabolism, and is a significant risk factor for insulin resistance and type 2 diabetes.

Treatment Of Disorders Of Insulin And Glucose Metabolism

Disorders in insulin and glucose metabolism can be treated using a variety of strategies, such as medication, lifestyle changes, and even surgery.

Diet and activity adjubstments are the cornerstone of diabetes management and prevention. A balanced diet that is high in fiber and low in added sugars and saturated fat can help control blood sugar levels and increase insulin sensitivity. Regular exercise can enhance insulin sensitivity and glycemic management. This includes both aerobic and resistance training.

A variety of drugs used in pharmacotherapy for diabetes aim to treat different elements of glucose metabolism, such as insulin production, insulin sensitivity, and glucose absorption. These drugs include injectable drugs like insulin and GLP-1 receptor agonists as well as oral hypoglycemic medicines like metformin and sulfonylureas.

By encouraging weight loss and enhancing insulin sensitivity, bariatric surgery, such as gastric bypass and sleeve gastrectomy, can help improve glucose metabolism in obese patients with type 2 diabetes.

Insulin is an important modulator of glucose absorption, gluconeogenesis, and glycogen formation, and it regulates the metabolism of glucose. Type 1 and type 2 diabetes, metabolic syndrome, and obesity are just a few of the metabolic illnesses that can develop as a result of insulin and glucose metabolism dysregulation. In order to get the best results, the treatment of abnormalities of insulin and glucose metabolism uses a variety of strategies, such as medication, surgery, and lifestyle changes.

Chapter 3

The Harms of High Blood Glucose

When the body has too much glucose (sugar) in the bloodstream, a condition known as hyperglycemia, also known as high blood sugar, develops. It is a typical side effect of diabetes, a chronic condition that affects millions of people globally. Numerous areas of a person's health, including their heart, kidneys, nerves, and eyes, might suffer from high blood sugar. We'll talk about the harmful effects of high blood sugar and how they influence the body in this essay.

The Harmful Effects of High Blood Glucose

1. Cardiovascular disease:
The cardiovascular system, which consists of the heart and blood arteries, can be negatively impacted by high blood glucose. High blood glucose levels have the potential to damage blood vessels and

result in atherosclerosis. The condition known as atherosclerosis causes the artery walls to thicken and constrict, which can reduce blood flow to the heart and other organs. Heart attacks, strokes, and other cardiovascular conditions may result from this.

2. Kidney disease:

The kidneys are in charge of removing waste from the blood through filtration. High blood glucose levels have the potential to harm the kidneys' tiny blood capillaries, resulting in diabetic nephropathy. In diabetic nephropathy, the kidneys become less effective at removing waste from the blood, which can result in kidney failure. Diabetic nephropathy is thought to affect 20–40% of adults with diabetes.

3. Nerve damage:

High blood sugar levels can potentially harm the neural system. High blood sugar levels can harm the nerves, which might result in neuropathy. Numbness, tingling, and pain in the hands and feet can result from neuropathy, a disorder where the nerves lose their capacity to transfer messages correctly. Additionally, it may result in digestive issues like nausea, vomiting, and diarrhea.

4. Eye disease:

Having high blood sugar might also harm your eyes. High blood sugar levels can harm the blood vessels in the eyes, resulting in diabetic retinopathy. In diabetic retinopathy, the blood vessels in the retina deteriorate, which can cause blindness and vision loss. According to estimates, 40–45% of patients with diabetes develop diabetic retinopathy to some extent.

5. Poor wound healing:

Wound healing can also be harmed by high blood glucose levels. Blood flow to the wound may be reduced when blood glucose levels are high, which may impede the healing process. Additionally, it may weaken the immune system, which could make infections more likely. For diabetics who are prone to foot ulcers and other sorts of sores, this can be very problematic.

6. Enhanced risk of infections:

Infections are also more likely to occur when blood sugar levels are high. High blood sugar levels can weaken the immune system, making it more difficult for the body to fight against diseases. Additionally, it may promote the growth and reproduction of bacteria and other diseases. This could make it more likely that you'll develop skin infections, urinary tract infections, and other diseases.

7. Sexual dysfunction:

High blood sugar levels can also impair sexual performance. High blood sugar levels can harm the nerves and blood vessels in the vaginal region, which can cause erectile dysfunction and other sexual issues. In addition, it can lower libido and sexual desire, which can be detrimental to one's quality of life.

8. Impairment of cognition:

High blood sugar levels can also have a detrimental effect on cognitive function. High blood glucose levels can affect the brain's blood flow, which can cause cognitive impairment. Additionally, it can harm the brain's nerves, which can cause memory loss, concentration issues, and other cognitive issues. For older persons with diabetes, who may already be at heightened risk for cognitive deterioration, this can be particularly problematic.

9. Mental health:

Having high blood sugar can also be detrimental to one's mental health. High blood sugar levels can result in irritation, exhaustion, and mood swings. It may also raise one's risk of developing depression and anxiety, both of which can be detrimental to one's quality of life. For those with diabetes, controlling blood glucose levels with food, exercise, and medication can assist to improve mental health outcomes.

10. Pregnancy complications:

High blood sugar levels can also have a detrimental effect on the course of a pregnancy. High blood glucose levels can raise the risk of difficulties for both the mother and the unborn child during pregnancy. Premature birth, gestational diabetes, and preeclampsia can result from it. Additionally, it may increase the baby's risk of having birth abnormalities and other problems.

Treatment and Prevention:

Through a combination of lifestyle modifications and medication interventions, the harmful effects of high blood glucose can be avoided and addressed.

Maintaining a balanced diet, exercising frequently, and abstaining from smoking and excessive alcohol consumption are all lifestyle modifications that can help control blood sugar levels and lower the risk of problems. Blood glucose levels can be managed and the risk of problems decreased with medical interventions such as insulin therapy and other drugs.

For persons with diabetes, routine blood glucose monitoring is crucial for managing and preventing high blood sugar levels. Diabetes patients should collaborate with their medical team to create a treatment strategy that addresses their unique requirements and objectives. This could involve taking drugs, altering one's lifestyle, and having regular checkups with the doctor.

High blood sugar, or hyperglycemia, can have detrimental effects on a person's heart, kidneys, nerves, eyes, wound healing, infections, sexual function, cognitive function, mental health, and pregnancy outcomes, among other areas of a person's health. However, these undesirable effects can be avoided and controlled with good management. Along with medications and routine doctor visits, lifestyle modifications including eating a nutritious diet and exercising frequently can help manage blood glucose levels. In order to avoid and manage high blood glucose levels and lower the risk of complications, it is crucial for individuals with diabetes to collaborate with their healthcare team to design a treatment plan that suits their unique requirements and objectives.

High Blood Glucose-related Health Risks

Hyperglycemia, or high blood sugar, is a condition where there is an abnormally high level of glucose in the blood. Although it is frequently linked to diabetes, this disorder can also affect those without the disease. Having high blood sugar levels carries a number of health hazards that may have varying effects on the body. In this book, we'll talk about the dangers of having high blood sugar and how to avoid them.

What causes high blood sugar?

It's critical to comprehend what high blood glucose is and how it impacts the body before delving into the health hazards linked to it. Blood glucose, sometimes referred to as blood sugar, is the body's cells' main source of energy. It comes from the food we eat and travels through the bloodstream to the cells. By enabling glucose to enter the cells, where it may be used for energy, the pancreatic hormone insulin helps control blood sugar levels.

High blood glucose levels occur in diabetics because the body either doesn't create enough insulin or doesn't utilise it properly. However, stress, illness, some drugs, consuming an excessive amount of sugar or refined carbs, or other factors can also cause high blood glucose levels in persons who do not have diabetes.

High Blood Glucose Risks for Your Health

There are a number of health hazards associated with high blood sugar levels, including both immediate and long-term consequences. The following are some of the most typical health hazards linked to high blood sugar:

1.Diabetes ketone bodies

When blood glucose levels rise to extremely high levels, a dangerous condition known as diabetic ketoacidosis (DKA) may develop. When the body begins to burn fat for fuel rather than glucose, producing ketones as a result, this disease develops. Because ketones are acidic, they can accumulate in the bloodstream and make it too acidic, which can be fatal.

DKA is most frequently observed in type 1 diabetics, although it can also happen in type 2 diabetics who are suffering from a serious sickness or infection. Shortness of breath, nausea, vomiting, stomach pain, and a fruity breath are all signs of DKA. Typically, hospitalization and insulin therapy are used to treat DKA.

2. hypoglycemia

Blood glucose levels that fall too low can cause hypoglycemia, often known as low blood sugar. This may occur if a diabetic consumes too much insulin or skips a meal. However, individuals without diabetes can also experience hypoglycemia, particularly those with liver or renal illness.

Shaking, dizziness, sweating, confusion, and a rapid heartbeat are all signs of hypoglycemia.

Hypoglycemia can cause convulsions or unconsciousness if it is not managed. Typically, a source of glucose, like juice or candy, is consumed as part of treatment for hypoglycemia.

3. Nerve Injury

Diabetic neuropathy is a disorder where high blood sugar levels damage the nerves. Although any region of the body might be affected by this ailment, the feet and legs are the most frequently affected. Numbness, tingling, and burning pain in the affected area are signs of diabetic neuropathy.

Diabetic neuropathy can eventually result in more severe problems like amputations and foot ulcers. In the case of gastroparesis, where the stomach takes longer to discharge food into the small intestine, it can also have an impact on the digestive system.

4. Eye Injury

Diabetic retinopathy, a disorder marked by high blood sugar levels, can potentially harm the eyes. The blood vessels in the retina become harmed in this illness, which can cause blindness or vision loss.

The signs of diabetic retinopathy can be hazy vision, floaters, or total blindness. Regular eye exams are crucial for diabetics in order to spot any early indications of diabetic retinopathy. Injections of medicine, laser surgery, or vitrectomy—a surgical operation that removes the gel-like substance from the eye—can all be used as treatments for diabetic retinopathy.

5. Kidney Injury

Diabetic nephropathy, a disorder marked by elevated blood sugar levels, can potentially harm the kidneys. Kidney function is reduced as a result of this disorder, which develops when the blood arteries in the kidneys are damaged.

Early signs of diabetic nephropathy may go unnoticed, but with time, the condition can progress to kidney failure, necessitating dialysis or kidney transplantation. Regular kidney function evaluations, such as blood tests to detect creatinine and urine examinations to assess protein levels, are recommended for diabetics.

6. Cardiovascular Illness

Cardiovascular disease, which encompasses illnesses like heart attack, stroke, and peripheral artery disease, can be brought on by high blood sugar levels. This is due to the fact that elevated blood glucose levels can harm blood vessels, increasing their susceptibility to plaque accumulation and constriction.

Cardiovascular disease is more likely to occur in persons with diabetes, but it can also happen to those without the condition if they have high blood sugar levels. It's critical to maintain a healthy lifestyle, which includes regular exercise, a nutritious diet, and quitting smoking, to lower the risk of cardiovascular disease.

7. Illnesses

The immune system may become weakened by high blood sugar levels, making it more difficult for the body to fight against diseases. Diabetes increases a person's risk of infection, including infections of the skin, urinary tract, and respiratory system.

People with diabetes must take particular care to avoid infections, including maintaining good cleanliness, avoiding close contact with ill people, and regularly monitoring blood glucose levels.

Keeping Blood Glucose Levels Low

Despite the fact that having high blood sugar levels might result in a number of health hazards, it is still feasible to prevent and treat this illness by making lifestyle adjustments and receiving medical care.

1. Eating well

One of the most crucial strategies to prevent high blood glucose levels is by eating a nutritious diet. This entails consuming moderate amounts of processed and sugary foods, as well as a variety of fruits, vegetables, whole grains, lean proteins, and healthy fats.

To avoid blood glucose levels rising or falling too low, it's also crucial to watch meal sizes and eat regularly throughout the day.

2. Consistent Exercise

Improved insulin sensitivity can make it simpler for the body to control blood glucose levels through regular exercise. At least 30 minutes of moderate-intensity exercise should be performed five days a week.

3. Medicine

To help control blood glucose levels, diabetics may need to take medicine, such as insulin or oral drugs. The optimal drug and dosage should be chosen in collaboration with a healthcare professional for each patient.

4. Checking Blood Sugar Levels

Regular blood glucose monitoring can aid diabetics in controlling their condition and avoiding complications. This can be achieved using continuous glucose monitoring (CGM) devices or self-monitoring of blood glucose using a glucometer.

5. Stress Control

It's crucial to manage stress through methods like deep breathing, meditation, or exercise because stress can raise blood glucose levels.

Numerous health hazards, including diabetic ketoacidosis, hypoglycemia, damage to the nerves, eyes, kidneys, and cardiovascular system, can be brought on by high blood sugar levels. However, lifestyle modifications, medication, and monitoring can help prevent and manage high blood sugar levels.

To maintain their blood glucose levels and avoid problems, people with diabetes should work closely with their healthcare professional to create a specific treatment plan. This can entail making adjustments to their eating and exercise routines, taking medication, and routinely checking their blood glucose levels.

The Relationship Between Chronic Diseases and High Blood Glucose

Hyperglycemia, or high blood sugar levels, is a medical disorder that develops when the bloodstream contains an excessive amount of glucose. Diabetes, a chronic disease that affects millions of individuals worldwide, is typically linked to this condition. However, other variables including stress, sickness, and medicine can also contribute to elevated blood sugar levels. Chronic illnesses and other serious health problems can result from persistently high blood glucose levels. The relationship between chronic diseases and high blood glucose levels will be discussed in this book.

Long-term health issues known as chronic diseases are those that last longer than three months and are typically brought on by a combination of genetic, environmental, and lifestyle factors. Cardiovascular disorders, cancer, chronic respiratory illnesses, and diabetes are only a few examples of the chronic diseases that are the main cause of mortality and disability globally. High blood sugar levels can seriously harm the body's essential organs, including the heart, kidneys, eyes, and nerves. They are a major risk factor for chronic diseases.

Diabetes is a chronic condition marked by elevated blood sugar levels brought on by the body's inability to make or use insulin properly. Diabetes is a major cause of death and disability that affects millions of people globally. The International Diabetes Federation estimates that 463 million people worldwide had diabetes in 2019; by 2045, this figure is expected to reach 700 million. Diabetes is a main cause of blindness, renal failure, and lower limb amputations as well as a significant risk factor for cardiovascular disorders like heart attacks and stroke.

It is well accepted that there is a connection between high blood glucose levels and chronic diseases, and that hyperglycemia plays a role in the onset and progression of many conditions. High blood sugar levels can harm the body through a number of ways, including oxidative stress, inflammation, and the production of advanced glycation end-products (AGEs).

When the body's capacity to neutralize free radicals and the generation of free radicals are out of balance, oxidative stress results. Free radicals are unstable chemicals that can harm cells and have a role in the emergence of chronic conditions like diabetes, heart disease, and cancer. Oxidative stress can result from high blood glucose levels since they can boost the body's generation of free radicals and decrease its capacity to fight them. Inflammation, DNA damage, and cellular malfunction can all be caused by oxidative stress, which can harm cells and tissues in the body.

The body's natural response to damage or illness is inflammation, which is crucial for the healing process. On the other hand, persistent inflammation can cause tissue damage and play a role in the emergence of chronic conditions like diabetes, cardiovascular disease, and cancer. Because high blood sugar levels activate immune cells like macrophages and release pro-inflammatory cytokines, they can lead to chronic inflammation. Chronic inflammation can harm the body's cells and tissues and speed up the onset and progression of chronic illnesses.

When glucose interacts with body proteins, cross-linked proteins are created that can damage the function of the proteins. These cross-linked proteins are known as advanced glycation end-products (AGEs). Diabetes patients have high amounts of AGEs, which are thought to have a role in the development of chronic illnesses. The function of many human tissues, including the kidneys, eyes, and nerves, can be hampered by the accumulation of AGEs. Additionally, AGEs can stimulate inflammation and activate immune cells like macrophages, which can cause tissue damage and the emergence of chronic illnesses.

Heart and blood vessel problems include coronary artery disease, heart failure, and stroke are among the chronic diseases known as cardiovascular diseases. About 31% of all deaths worldwide are caused by cardiovascular illnesses, which are the main cause of death worldwide. It is thought that hyperglycemia plays a role in the onset and progression of cardiovascular diseases and is a substantial risk factor for these illnesses.

Damage to the blood arteries is one way that high blood sugar levels can cause cardiovascular problems. Oxidative stress and inflammation brought on by high blood sugar levels can harm the endothelial cells that line the blood vessels. Damage to blood vessels can result in plaque buildup, which can restrict arteries and limit blood flow to important organs including the heart and brain. Additionally, narrowed arteries have the potential to burst, resulting in blood clots that can cause heart attacks and strokes.

By encouraging the production of advanced glycation end-products (AGEs), high blood glucose levels can also contribute to cardiovascular disorders. Blood flow to crucial organs including the heart and brain can be diminished as a result of AGE buildup in blood vessels that compromises their ability to operate. Inflammation and immune cell activation caused by AGEs can result in tissue damage and the emergence of cardiovascular illnesses.

High blood glucose levels are thought to aid in the onset and progression of kidney disease, which is at high risk for development in people with diabetes. The body's fluid balance is controlled by the kidneys, which also filter waste from the blood. Kidney blood flow may be diminished as a result of kidney blood vessel damage brought on by diabetes, which also affects kidney function. Additionally, oxidative stress and inflammation brought on by high blood glucose levels can harm kidney tissue and result in the onset of renal disease.

Diabetes patients can develop diabetic nephropathy, which is another name for diabetic kidney disease. Damage to the kidney's blood arteries causes impaired kidney function and an accumulation of waste products in the blood, which is the hallmark of diabetic nephropathy. End-stage kidney disease, which necessitates dialysis or kidney transplantation, is frequently brought on by diabetic nephropathy.

Having high blood sugar levels might also increase the risk of developing eye conditions like diabetic retinopathy. A consequence of diabetes called diabetic retinopathy affects the blood vessels in the retina, impairing vision and even causing blindness.

High blood sugar levels can harm the retina's blood vessels, resulting in decreased blood flow and the emergence of brand-new, aberrant blood vessels. These aberrant blood arteries have the potential to leak blood and fluid into the retina, resulting in blindness and vision loss.

Diabetic neuropathy, a complication of diabetes, can harm the nerves. Chronic diabetic neuropathy damages the nerves in the feet and legs and causes pain, numbness, and decreased sensation. High blood sugar levels can damage and impair nerve function by causing oxidative stress and inflammation in the nerves. Additionally, muscle weakness and decreased balance brought on by diabetic neuropathy might increase the risk of fractures and falls.

chronic disorders like cardiovascular problems, kidney problems, eye problems, and nerve damage are all significantly increased by high blood glucose levels. Blood glucose levels that are too high can harm the body's essential organs, resulting in tissue damage, inflammation, and reduced function. Oxidative stress, inflammation, and the production of advanced glycation end products are some of the mechanisms by which elevated blood sugar levels cause chronic illnesses. In order to lower the risk of chronic diseases and enhance the health of diabetics, high blood glucose levels must be prevented and managed. Changing your lifestyle to include regular exercise, a balanced diet, and weight management will help you manage your blood sugar levels and lower your chance of developing chronic diseases. The risk of developing chronic diseases can be decreased by managing high blood glucose levels with medications like insulin and oral hypoglycemic medicines. It's critical to collaborate closely with healthcare professionals to create a personalized management plan that takes into account the specific requirements of each diabetic person.

High Blood Glucose's Financial Costs

Hyperglycemia, or high blood sugar, is a condition where the blood sugar level exceeds the usual range. This illness is widespread and a serious public health issue in both industrialized and developing nations. Numerous consequences, such as cardiovascular illness, kidney disease, nerve damage, and blindness, are linked to high blood sugar levels. These issues have a huge financial impact on people, families, and healthcare systems. The cost of having high blood sugar, its effects on people and society, and potential treatments will all be covered in this book.

High blood sugar has a significant financial cost that impacts people, families, and society as a whole. Medical costs including hospital stays, prescription drugs, and surgical procedures are included in the direct costs of having high blood sugar. These expenses are frequently substantial, especially for people who need continuous care for issues brought on by high blood sugar. For instance, the price of insulin, a drug frequently used to treat high blood sugar, has climbed dramatically in recent years, putting a strain on individuals' finances and the healthcare system.

High blood sugar levels may have major indirect consequences, such as missed productivity and a lower quality of life. High blood sugar sufferers could have issues that make it difficult for them to work or go about their regular lives. People who have diabetic retinopathy, a side effect of high blood sugar that can result in blindness, may find it challenging to perform activities that call for good visual acuity, including driving or reading. Loss of income and a decline in quality of life for the individual and their family are potential outcomes.

High blood sugar also has an economic cost to society as a whole. The cost of treating issues brought on by high blood sugar, which can be quite considerable, falls on healthcare systems. For instance, a 2012 study from the United States indicated that $245 billion was spent annually on diabetes-related healthcare. In the upcoming years, it is anticipated that this cost would rise dramatically, putting a heavy burden on healthcare systems and taxpayers.

Effects of High Blood Glucose on People

High blood sugar levels have a substantial effect on people and may have negative health and psychological effects. Numerous consequences, including cardiovascular illness, kidney disease, nerve damage, and blindness, can occur in people with high blood sugar. These issues may prevent the person from carrying out regular tasks and may necessitate continuing medical care.

The psychological effects of high blood sugar are as substantial and can include depressive, anxious, and socially isolated sensations. People with high blood sugar may experience stigma or judgment as a result of their disease, which can cause them to feel ashamed or embarrassed. These psychological impacts may make it harder for the person to carry out daily tasks and may lower their quality of life as a whole.

The Effects of High Blood Glucose on Families

High blood sugar levels have an effect on the individual as well as their family. Families of people with high blood sugar may face financial hardship due to the expense of medical care and lost wages. Due to the psychological repercussions of high blood glucose on the individual, they could also experience emotional stress. If they are unable to offer sufficient support, family members may feel anxious or guilty about their failure to take care of the person.

Healthcare System Effects of High Blood Glucose:

Healthcare systems are heavily burdened by high blood sugar, especially in developed nations where the illness is prevalent. The cost of treating complications brought on by high blood sugar, such as hospitalizations, surgeries, and drugs, must be covered by healthcare systems. These expenses may make it more difficult for healthcare systems to treat additional patients because they can be rather high.

Possibilities for Reducing the Economic Cost of High Blood Glucose
The financial burden of high blood sugar has a number of potential solutions. These remedies consist of:

1.Prevention

One of the best ways to lessen the financial toll of this condition is to prevent excessive blood glucose. This can be done by implementing public health programs that encourage healthy lifestyle choices like regular exercise, a balanced diet, and weight control. Furthermore, early intervention and the development of fully-blown high blood glucose can be prevented through screening programs that identify those with pre-diabetes or at risk of acquiring the condition.

2. Improved Blood Glucose Management

The financial cost of high blood sugar might also be lessened with improved management. Better access to healthcare services, such as medical treatment, drugs, and monitoring tools, can help with this. Technology can also facilitate remote monitoring of high blood glucose levels and enhance access to care. Examples of this include telemedicine and mobile health apps.

3. Taking Social Determinants of Health into Account

High blood sugar can develop and progress due to social determinants of health such poverty, food insecurity, and lack of access to healthcare. By addressing these social variables, high blood sugar can be avoided, and those who already have it can experience better results. Initiatives that support food access, healthcare services, and economic stability might all fall under this category.

4. Innovation and research

Additionally important in easing the financial burden of high blood sugar is research and innovation. This may involve the creation of novel drugs and medical advancements that enhance the results for people with high blood sugar. Research on the root causes of high blood sugar and its side effects can also help to guide preventative and management plans.

High blood sugar levels are a serious public health issue that have a large financial impact on people, families, and healthcare systems. The disorder has significant direct and indirect costs and can make it difficult for people to carry out everyday tasks and lower their quality of life. To lessen the financial burden of high blood sugar, there are a number of potential solutions, such as prevention, better management, addressing social determinants of health, and research and innovation. To improve outcomes for people with high blood glucose and lessen the financial burden this condition places on society as a whole, these solutions call for a concerted effort from individuals, healthcare professionals, and politicians.

Chapter 4

Promising Research on The Glucose Breakthrough

The term "glucose breakthrough" refers to exciting studies that have been done on the metabolism of glucose and how it affects general health. This study has shed new light on how blood glucose influences several facets of human health and underlined the need of maintaining healthy blood glucose levels.

This research has shown significant promise in the treatment and prevention of diabetes, to name one area. Diabetes is a chronic disease that affects millions of people worldwide and is defined by increased blood glucose levels. The Glucose Breakthrough has sparked the creation of novel diabetes therapies, including drugs that focus on particular facets of glucose metabolism.

The Glucose Breakthrough has made clear how important glucose is to other aspects of health in addition to diabetes. For instance, studies have shown that elevated glucose levels can raise the risk of cardiovascular disease and also have a role in dementia and cognitive decline. On the other hand, preserving normal blood sugar levels can aid in preventing these ailments and enhancing general health and wellbeing.

Utilizing technology to monitor and control blood glucose levels is one of the intriguing research areas being investigated by the Glucose Breakthrough. Continuous glucose monitoring (CGM) devices, as an illustration, can offer real-time input on glucose levels, enabling people to make wise decisions regarding their dietary, physical activity, and prescription regimes. This technology has the potential to transform the treatment of diabetes and enhance outcomes for millions of patients worldwide.

human knowledge of how glucose affects human health and how to work to maintain appropriate blood glucose levels has advanced significantly as a result of the Glucose Breakthrough. We can create new methods for avoiding and treating diabetes and advancing general health and wellbeing by using the most recent studies and technological advancements.

The utilization of dietary and lifestyle changes to control blood glucose levels is one potential area of research in the Glucose Breakthrough. For instance, research suggests that consuming a diet high in fiber and low in simple carbohydrates can help to control blood sugar levels and lower the chance of developing diabetes. Regular exercise has also been proven to enhance insulin sensitivity and glucose metabolism, which can aid in the management and prevention of diabetes.

The function of gut bacteria in glucose metabolism is another topic of study in the Glucose Breakthrough. Studies have revealed that changes in the gut microbiota can alter blood glucose levels and that the gut microbiota's composition can affect how glucose is metabolized. New probiotic and prebiotic therapies that can aid in regulating gut flora and enhancing glucose metabolism have been developed as a result of this.

Overall, the glucose breakthrough has revealed fresh information about the intricate connection between glucose and our health and has opened up fascinating new directions for investigation and therapy. We can create innovative methods for preventing and controlling diabetes and advance global health and welfare by continuing to build on this study.

The Glucose Breakthrough has also showed promise in the creation of fresh drugs that focus on particular facets of glucose metabolism. For instance, new drugs have been created that target sodium-glucose cotransporter-2 (SGLT2), a protein in the kidneys that reabsorbs glucose. These drugs lower blood glucose levels by preventing the reabsorption of glucose, allowing it to be discharged in the urine, and doing so. Glucagon-like peptide-1 (GLP-1), a hormone that promotes insulin secretion and curbs hunger, is the target of additional drugs. These drugs can encourage weight loss and aid to control blood sugar levels.

The Glucose Breakthrough has also stimulated the creation of fresh methods for controlling and monitoring blood sugar levels. New insulin pumps and delivery systems have also been created, which can offer more accurate and automated insulin delivery in addition to continuous glucose monitoring devices. This can lessen the strain of managing diabetes and enhance the outcomes for those who have the disease.

Finally, the necessity of customized methods to glucose management has been emphasized by the Glucose Breakthrough. Although there are broad recommendations for keeping blood glucose levels in a healthy range, each person has a different metabolism, so what works for one person may not work for another. Healthcare professionals can assist people in optimizing their glucose levels and enhancing their general health and wellbeing by using a tailored approach to glucose management.

In conclusion, the Glucose Breakthrough has advanced our knowledge of how our bodies use glucose and how that knowledge affects our health. We can create new methods for avoiding and treating diabetes and advancing general health and wellbeing by using the most recent studies and technological advancements. We may anticipate future innovations and advancements in glucose management as we build on this research, which will enhance results for people all across the world.

Diets With A Low GI And Glucose Regulation

In order to control blood sugar levels and lessen the risk of developing Type 2 diabetes, the Low Glycemic Index (GI) Diet emphasizes foods with a lower glycemic index. The glycemic index is a measure of how quickly a food can cause an individual's blood sugar levels to rise. Blood sugar levels quickly rise after eating foods with a high GI, while levels rise more slowly and gradually after eating foods with a low GI. We will talk about the Low GI Diet and its advantages for glucose regulation in this book.

Knowing The Glycemic Index:

The rate at which meal carbs are broken down into glucose in the blood is gauged using the Glycemic Index (GI) scale. The scale has a range of 0 to 100, with 100 representing the best result. High glycemic index (GI) foods are rapidly metabolized and assimilated, leading to a steep increase in blood glucose levels. Foods with a low GI score, on the other hand, are digested and absorbed more gradually, causing a slower increase in blood sugar levels.

A food's glycemic index is influenced by a number of elements, such as the kind of carbohydrate it contains, how much fiber it has, and how it was prepared. A baked potato, for instance, has a high glycemic index due to the quantity of starch it contains, which is quickly converted to glucose. The glycemic index is lower if the potato is consumed with the skin, which has fiber.

Glucose Control Benefits of a Low Glycemic Index Diet:

Numerous advantages for glucose control of the low glycemic index diet have been demonstrated, including:

1. Better Blood Sugar Control:

Diabetics can better control their blood sugar levels by selecting foods with a lower glycemic index. Foods with a lower glycemic index raise blood sugar levels more gradually and slowly, which helps lessen the likelihood of blood sugar spikes and crashes.

2. Lessened Insulin Resistance:

Insulin resistance is a condition in which the body loses its sensitivity to the hormone insulin, which helps control blood sugar levels. A common contributing factor to the onset of Type 2 diabetes is insulin resistance. A Low GI diet can enhance insulin sensitivity and lessen insulin resistance, according to studies.

3. Lessening the chance of Type 2 Diabetes:

It has been demonstrated that a Low GI diet lowers the chance of developing Type 2 diabetes. In contrast to people who had a diet with a higher glycemic index, those who consumed a diet with a lower glycemic index had a lower chance of acquiring Type 2 diabetes, according to a study that was published in the American Journal of Clinical Nutrition.

4. Enhanced Cardiovascular Health:

It has also been demonstrated that a low GI diet enhances cardiovascular health. According to research in the Journal of the American Medical Association, people who followed a low glycemic index diet had lower levels of LDL cholesterol, a form of cholesterol Having a connection to a greater probability of developing heart disease.

Dietary Items With A Low Glycemic Index:
The Low GI Diet focuses on picking meals with a lower glycemic index rather than being low in carbohydrates. Included in a low GI diet are the following foods:

1.Whole Grains:
Refined grains have a higher glycemic index than whole grains. Brown rice, quinoa, and whole wheat bread are some instances of whole grains.

2. Fruits:
Compared to processed carbohydrates and sweets, most fruits have a lower glycemic index. Fruits like citrus, berries, and apples are terrific options.

3. Vegetables:

Non-starchy vegetables with a low glycemic index include leafy greens, broccoli, and cauliflower.

4. Legumes:

Chickpeas, lentils, and beans are nutritious sources of protein with low glycemic indexes.

5. Nuts and Seeds:

Nuts and seeds have a low glycemic index and are a wonderful source of healthy fats. A few examples are almonds, walnuts, and chia seeds.

6. Dairy:

Milk, yoghourt, and cheese are examples of dairy items with low glycemic indexes that can be incorporated into a low glycemic index diet.

7. Protein:

Lean protein foods with a low glycemic index, like chicken, fish, and tofu, can help control blood sugar levels.

Dietary Avoidances for Low Glycemic Index:

Foods to limit or avoid when following a low GI diet include:

1.Refined Carbohydrates:

Because they have a high glycemic index, refined carbohydrates like white bread, white rice, and pasta should be avoided or consumed in moderation.

2. Sugary meals:

Sugary meals should be avoided because they have a high glycemic index, including soda, candy, and cookies.

3. Processed Foods:

Because they frequently contain refined carbs, processed foods like chips, crackers, and snack bars should be avoided or consumed in moderation.

4. High-Fat Foods:

A Low GI diet should avoid high-fat foods such fried foods and fatty meats.

Follow These Tips for a Low Glycemic Index Diet:

1. Select whole, unprocessed foods:

Reducing the glycemic index of your diet is simple when you select entire, unprocessed foods. Choose fruit instead of a sugary snack, for instance, or brown rice instead of white rice.

2. Include fibre:

Fibre can aid in reducing the rate at which glucose enters the bloodstream. Include foods high in fibre in your diet, such as fruits, vegetables, and whole grains.

3. Consume smaller, more frequent meals:

Eating more frequent, smaller meals can help reduce blood sugar increases and crashes. Eat three to four meals each day, including one with a source of fibre and protein.

4. Keep an eye on portion sizes:

A Low GI diet does not necessitate tight portion restriction, but it is still necessary to keep an eye on portion proportions. Even foods with a low glycemic index can raise blood sugar levels when consumed in excess.

5. Maintain consistency:

Adhering to a Low GI Diet requires consistency. At each meal and snack, strive to choose healthy options, and make an effort to maintain a regular eating pattern.

A dietary strategy known as the Low Glycemic Index Diet focuses on selecting foods with a lower glycemic index. This can enhance cardiovascular health, lessen the risk of Type 2 diabetes, reduce insulin resistance, and regulate blood sugar levels. You can adhere to a Low GI Diet and improve your glucose control by including whole, unprocessed foods, fibre, and protein in your diet while avoiding refined carbohydrates, sugary meals, and processed foods. Keep an eye on your portion sizes and stick to your healthy habits. Before making any dietary or exercise regimen adjustments, speak with a healthcare practitioner.

Glucose Regulation And Exercise

Regular physical activity is crucial for maintaining a healthy way of life. Regular exercise, together with a healthy diet, can help avoid chronic conditions including type 2 diabetes, heart disease, and obesity. Exercise has several advantages, including helping people manage their weight and improving their cardiovascular and mental health as well as their energy levels. Regular exercise has also been demonstrated to help people with and without diabetes better regulate their blood sugar. In this book, the relationship between exercise and glucose regulation will be examined, along with the mechanisms underlying it and the effects of various types and intensities of exercise.

Glucose Control

The main fuel for the body's cells is a form of sugar called glucose. In the form of glycogen, which may be broken down to release glucose into the bloodstream when needed, glucose is stored in the liver and muscles. Because glucose levels that are too high or too low can result in a number of health issues, maintaining glucose homeostasis is essential for good health in general.

Glucagon and Insulin

Two hormones, insulin and glucagon, work together to control blood glucose levels in the body. The pancreas produces insulin in response to escalating blood glucose levels. Insulin influences how quickly glucose is absorbed from the bloodstream and stored as glycogen in the liver, muscles, and fat cells. In addition to preventing glucose production and release from the liver, insulin also promotes glucose homeostasis.

On the other hand, the pancreas releases glucagon in reaction to decreasing blood glucose levels. When glucose acts on the liver, it encourages the release of glucose into the bloodstream and the breakdown of glycogen. By doing so, hypoglycemia is avoided and blood glucose levels are raised.

Exercise and Blood Sugar Control

Regular exercise has been demonstrated to help people with and without diabetes better regulate their blood sugar. By increasing muscle glucose uptake and reducing liver glucose production, exercise lowers blood glucose levels. The ability of insulin to enhance glucose uptake and storage in the liver, muscle, and fat cells is also increased by exercise.

Efficacy Mechanisms

Exercise's positive benefits on glucose regulation are mediated by a variety of intricate processes. Increased muscle glucose uptake is one of the main mechanisms. Muscle contractions during exercise promote the uptake of glucose into the muscle cells from the circulation. The glucose transporter GLUT4, which is insulin-independent, does this by moving to the surface of muscle cells in response to muscular contractions.

The cellular energy sensor AMP-activated protein kinase (AMPK), which controls glucose metabolism, is similarly stimulated by exercise. AMPK encourages the muscles' uptake of glucose while preventing the liver's ability to produce it. The breakdown of fatty acids in muscle, which can be used as an energy source during exercise, is also sped up by AMPK.

Improved insulin sensitivity is another mechanism behind the positive benefits of exercise on glucose regulation. Exercise has been demonstrated to boost insulin receptor expression on the surface of muscle cells, facilitating insulin's ability to promote glucose uptake and storage. Exercise also enhances the activity of various signaling pathways, including the Akt and mTOR pathways, which are crucial for insulin signaling.

Effects of Exercise Intensity and Type

Depending on the kind and level of exercise, the effect on glucose regulation may differ. Exercise that increases muscle glucose uptake and increases insulin sensitivity, such running or cycling, has been found to enhance glucose regulation. By boosting muscle development and enhancing insulin sensitivity, resistance training, such as weightlifting, can also help with glucose regulation.

Exercise intensity can also affect how well glucose is regulated. It has been demonstrated that high-intensity interval training (HIIT) is particularly effective at enhancing glucose regulation, probably as a result of its capacity to raise AMPK activation and muscle uptake of glucose. The advantages of HIIT may, however, be outweighed by the risk of increased bodily stress, which, if not done appropriately, might result in overtraining and injury.

Walking, on the other hand, may not have the same major effect on glucose regulation as more intense exercise. Low-intensity exercise, however, may be more enduring for people with reduced mobility or fitness levels and still be good for general health.

Exercise Timing and Duration

Exercise duration and timing can have an effect on how glucose is regulated. Exercise has been demonstrated to be especially beneficial for enhancing glucose management when done postprandially, or right after eating. This is due to the fact that exercise at this time can encourage the muscles' uptake of glucose and prevent the liver's creation of glucose, both of which contribute to a reduction in blood glucose levels.

Exercise length can have an effect on how well glucose is regulated. Exercise that lasts only 10 to

15 minutes has been demonstrated to help type 2 diabetics better control their blood sugar levels. In people without diabetes, longer exercise sessions of 30 to 60 minutes may be required to improve glucose control. It's crucial to remember that exercise of any kind helps improve glucose control and general health.

Diabetes Type 2 and Exercise

An essential part of controlling type 2 diabetes is regular exercise. By boosting muscle glucose absorption and enhancing insulin sensitivity, exercise can enhance glucose regulation. Exercise can also aid with weight control, which is crucial for managing and avoiding type 2 diabetes.

The American Diabetes Association advises people with type 2 diabetes to exercise for at least 150 minutes per week, spaced out across at least three days, and to avoid going more than two days straight without exercising. A minimum of two to three times a week of resistance training is also advised, with an emphasis on all the major muscle groups.

Diabetes Type 1 and Exercise

People with type 1 diabetes can also benefit from exercise, while it can be difficult to control blood sugar levels when working out. Blood glucose levels can decline after exercise, especially for those who take insulin or other blood glucose-lowering drugs. However, people with type 1 diabetes can safely exercise and improve their glucose regulation with the right planning and supervision.

It is advised that people with type 1 diabetes check their blood sugar levels before, during, and after physical activity. If necessary, they should change their insulin dosage or carbohydrate intake. To avoid hypoglycemia, it may also be beneficial to eat a snack before and/or during exercise. To avoid hypoglycemia after exercise, people with type 1 diabetes may also need to change their insulin dosages.

Regular exercise can help people with and without diabetes better regulate their blood sugar.It is fundamental to living a healthy lifestyle. Exercise increases insulin sensitivity, enhances muscle glucose absorption, and reduces hepatic glucose production. Exercise type, intensity, timing, and duration can all have an effect on how glucose is regulated. Exercise is especially crucial for controlling type 2 diabetes, while it can also be helpful for people with type 1 diabetes with the right planning and supervision.

Medicines For Treating High Blood Glucose

To avoid long-term diabetic problems like heart disease, renal failure, nerve damage, and blindness, managing high blood glucose is crucial. The use of medications, either alone or in conjunction with other lifestyle changes including diet and exercise, is essential in the management of high blood glucose. We will cover the many drugs used to treat high blood sugar in this book, along with their methods of action, adverse effects, and warnings.

Types of Drugs for Treating High Blood Sugar

For the treatment of high blood sugar, there are numerous pharmacological options available, and each one has a unique mechanism of action. The primary categories of drugs are:

1.Insulin

The pancreas secretes the hormone insulin, which lowers blood sugar levels by assisting the body's cells in absorbing glucose. High blood glucose levels are caused by poor insulin synthesis or activity in diabetic patients. To complement or replace the body's natural insulin, insulin is injected into the body during insulin therapy.

There are various insulin varieties, including:

- Insulin with a rapid onset of action (RAI) has its greatest effect in roughly an hour after injection. In order to prevent postprandial (after-meal) glucose increases, it is often administered before meals.

- Insulin with a short half-life: This kind of insulin begins to function within 30 minutes of injection and reaches its peak in around 2-3 hours. To prevent postprandial glucose rises, it is often taken before meals.

- Insulin with an intermediate half-life begins to function between two and four hours after injection and peaks between four and twelve hours later. In order to give basal (background) insulin coverage, it is normally taken twice day.

- Long-acting insulin: This kind of insulin has a reasonably flat and steady impact for up to 24 hours after injection and begins to work within 1-2 hours. In order to cover the need for basal insulin, it is normally administered once day.

- Combination insulin: This kind of insulin combines both long- and rapid-acting forms of the hormone in a single injection. In order to cover both basal and prandial (mealtime) insulin, it is often taken twice daily.

When using insulin therapy, blood glucose levels must be closely monitored and the insulin dose must be changed in response to things like diet, activity, illness, and stress. Hypoglycemia (low blood sugar) can result after insulin therapy if too much insulin is administered or the timing of the injections is not appropriate for the body's requirements.

2. Medicines taken orally

medicines given orally to reduce blood sugar levels are referred to as oral medicines. Oral drugs come in a variety of forms, including:

- The most often recommended oral diabetic medicine is metformin. It functions by lowering hepatic glucose synthesis and raising muscle cell sensitivity to insulin. It can be used alone or in conjunction with other drugs and does not result in hypoglycemia.

- Sulfonylureas: Sulfonylureas increase the production of insulin from the pancreas, reducing blood sugar levels. They are commonly used by persons with type 2 diabetes who produce enough insulin and are at risk for hypoglycemia.

- Meglitinides: Meglitinides likewise increase pancreatic insulin production, but their duration of action is less than that of sulfonylureas. They are commonly used before to meals in order to reduce postprandial glucose rises, although they can also result in hypoglycemia.

- DPP-4 inhibitors: DPP-4 inhibitors function by preventing the enzyme DPP-4 from degrading the hormone incretin. Blood glucose levels are decreased and insulin production is stimulated by incretin. DPP-4 inhibitors do not result in hypoglycemia and can be used alone or in conjunction with other drugs.

- GLP-1 receptor agonists: GLP-1 receptor agonists stimulate the secretion of insulin by imitating the effects of incretin. Additionally, they slow down stomach emptying, which aids in reducing postprandial glucose increases. GLP-1 receptor agonists do not result in hypoglycemia and can be taken alone or in conjunction with other drugs.

- SGLT2 inhibitors: SGLT2 inhibitors function by preventing the kidneys from reabsorbing glucose, which increases the excretion of glucose through the urine and lowers blood glucose levels. Additionally, they have positive benefits on weight and blood pressure. SGLT2 inhibitors can have an uncommon but dangerous side effect known as diabetic ketoacidosis (DKA), which can occur when they are administered alone or in conjunction with other drugs.

3. Medications for injection

drug that is provided via injection and lowers blood glucose levels is known as an injectable drug. Injectable drugs come in a variety of forms, including:

- GLP-1 receptor agonists: Depending on the drug, GLP-1 receptor agonists can be injected once a week or daily. They function by promoting the synthesis of insulin and acting like incretin. Additionally, they slow down stomach emptying, which aids in reducing postprandial glucose increases. GLP-1 receptor agonists do not result in hypoglycemia and can be taken alone or in conjunction with other drugs.

- Amylin analogs: Amylin analogs are manufactured forms of the hormone amylin, which the pancreas also produces alongside insulin. Amylin aids in reducing blood sugar levels, suppressing hunger, and delaying gastric emptying. Analogs of amylin can be used with insulin and do not result in hypoglycemia.

- Insulin: As previously mentioned, insulin therapy can also be given by injection.

Medication Mechanisms of Action for Treating High Blood Glucose

The mechanisms of action of drugs used to treat high blood sugar vary depending on the drug.

Insulin therapy works by augmenting or replacing the body's natural insulin and assisting the body's cells in absorbing glucose. The timing of meals and exercise can be adjusted to accommodate the body's insulin requirements.

Different strategies are used by oral medicines to reduce blood sugar levels. Metformin acts by lowering hepatic glucose synthesis and raising muscle cell sensitivity to insulin. Meglitinides and sulfonylureas encourage the pancreas to produce more insulin. Incretin is broken down by the enzyme DPP-4, which is blocked by DPP-4 inhibitors. GLP-1 receptor agonists promote the secretion of insulin by simulating the effects of incretin. Inhibitors of SGLT2 stop the kidneys from reabsorption of glucose.

Similar mechanisms underlie the action of oral and injectable medicines. GLP-1 receptor agonists promote the secretion of insulin by simulating the effects of incretin. Amylin analogs work similarly to amylin in that they slow down stomach emptying, curb hunger, and regulate blood sugar levels.

Medication Side Effects and Precautions for Treating High Blood Glucose

Drugs used to treat high blood sugar might have negative effects, therefore care must be taken to use them safely and effectively.

If too much insulin is administered or if mealtimes or exercise sessions are not coordinated with insulin injection times, insulin therapy may result in hypoglycemia. Weight gain and adverse reactions at the injection site are additional side effects of insulin therapy.

The usage of oral drugs to treat high blood sugar might have negative side effects as well. The gastrointestinal adverse effects of metformin might include nausea, vomiting, and diarrhea. Meglitinides and sulfonylureas may result in hypoglycemia if excessive amounts of insulin are generated. GLP-1 receptor agonists and DPP-4 inhibitors can both produce gastrointestinal adverse effects like nausea and diarrhea. Urinary tract infections and diabetic ketoacidosis are both unusual side effects of SGLT2 inhibitors.

The injectable drugs used to treat high blood sugar might also have negative side effects. Constipation and diarrhea are two gastrointestinal adverse effects that GLP-1 receptor agonists can produce. Analogs of amylin when combined with insulin can result in nausea and hypoglycemia.

A balanced diet and exercise routine should be followed in addition to routinely checking blood glucose levels and modifying medication dosages as necessary when using drugs to manage high blood sugar. If side effects develop or blood glucose levels are not sufficiently controlled, some drugs may need to be changed or stopped.

Considerations to Make When Selecting Drugs to Treat High Blood Glucose

When selecting drugs to treat high blood sugar, there are a number of things to take into account, including:

- Effectiveness: A key factor to take into account is how well a medicine lowers blood sugar levels. Some patient populations may respond better to some drugs than others.

- Safety: Another crucial factor to take into account is a drug's safety profile. other medications may not be suitable for patients with particular medical conditions and other medications may carry a higher risk of side effects than others.

- Cost: For many patients, a medication's price is a crucial factor. Some prescriptions can cost more than others, and some might have insurance coverage while others would not.

- Convenience: Another crucial factor is a medication's ease of use. While some medications must be administered numerous times each day through injection, others can be taken just once or once a week.

- Patient preference: The preference of the patient for a drug is also crucial. Others may prefer drugs that do not cause hypoglycemia. Some patients may prefer oral meds over injectable treatments.

Controlling high blood sugar levels is a crucial part of managing diabetes. Oral medicines and injectable drugs can both be used to treat high blood sugar levels; each has a unique mechanism of action and negative effects. When selecting drugs to treat high blood sugar, factors like efficacy, safety, cost, and patient preference should be taken into account. To find the optimal pharmaceutical regimen for their particular needs, patients should consult carefully with their medical team.

Innovative Methods Of Managing Glucose

Millions of individuals throughout the world suffer from the chronic condition of diabetes. High blood glucose levels are one of its defining characteristics, and they can cause a variety of consequences, such as cardiovascular disease, kidney failure, blindness, and neuropathy. One of the most important parts of managing diabetes is controlling glucose. There is a need for creative techniques to improve the outcomes of glucose management, even while established approaches to glucose management, such as insulin therapy and lifestyle changes, have been successful in regulating blood glucose levels.

Significant progress has been made in the creation of fresh methods for managing glucose in recent years. These strategies include brand-new drugs, tools, and technologies that can assist patients in better controlling their blood sugar levels. This book will go through a few of these cutting-edge strategies for controlling glucose.

1.Continuous Glucose Monitoring

A relatively new technology called continuous glucose monitoring (CGM) has completely changed how people regulate their blood sugar levels. To detect glucose levels continually, CGM systems insert a tiny sensor just beneath the skin. Patients may monitor their blood sugar levels in real-time thanks to the sensor, which transmits glucose measurements to a receiver or smartphone.

Compared to conventional methods of self-monitoring blood glucose (SMBG), CGM systems offer more detailed information on glucose levels. They can identify glucose swings that SMBG might overlook and give patients greater knowledge about how different variables like diet and exercise can affect their blood glucose levels. Additionally, CGM can notify patients of hypo- and hyperglycemic episodes, enabling them to take the necessary action.

2. Open-Loop Systems

A potential new strategy for managing glucose is called a closed-loop system, which is also referred to as an artificial pancreas system. These devices establish a closed-loop system that can automatically change insulin dose based on blood glucose levels by integrating a CGM with an insulin pump. In order to forecast glucose changes and modify insulin dosing accordingly, the system uses algorithms.

It has been demonstrated that closed-loop devices enhance glucose regulation and lower the possibility of hypoglycemia. They are especially helpful for patients with type 1 diabetes or those who need intense insulin therapy and have trouble controlling their blood sugar levels.

3. Opponents of the glucagon-like peptide-1 (GLP-1) receptor

A relatively recent class of drugs known as GLP-1 receptor agonists has been found to enhance glycemic control outcomes. These drugs function by imitating GLP-1, a hormone that the intestine releases in response to meal intake. By promoting insulin production and preventing glucagon secretion, GLP-1 aids in controlling blood glucose levels.

Compared to conventional diabetic treatments, GLP-1 receptor agonists provide a number of advantages. They are linked to weight loss and have been demonstrated to enhance cardiovascular outcomes in diabetic individuals. In comparison to insulin therapy, they also have a lower risk of hypoglycemia.

4. Drugs that inhibit Sodium-Glucose Cotransporter-2 (SGLT2)

Another novel family of drugs that has been demonstrated to enhance glycemic control results is the SGLT2 inhibitors. These drugs function by preventing the kidneys from reabsorbing glucose, which causes an increase in the excretion of glucose through the urine.

SGLT2 inhibitors are superior to conventional diabetic treatments in a number of ways. They are linked to weight loss and have been demonstrated to enhance cardiovascular outcomes in diabetic individuals. In comparison to insulin therapy, they also have a lower risk of hypoglycemia.

5. Beta Cell Replacement

The goal of beta cell regeneration, a revolutionary strategy for controlling blood sugar, is to revive the pancreas' beta cells, which produce insulin. Stem cells, gene therapy, or other methods of regenerative medicine may be used to regenerate beta cells.

Although beta cell regeneration is still in its infancy, it has the potential to fundamentally alter how diabetes patients manage their blood sugar levels. Instead of only controlling diabetes with drugs and dietary changes, it may be feasible to reverse or cure disease by restoring beta cell function.

6. Therapies based on incretin

A group of medicines known as incretin-based therapies act by boosting the effects of GLP-1 and other incretin hormones. These drugs include glucagon-like peptide-1 receptor agonists (GLP-1 RAs) and dipeptidyl peptidase-4 (DPP-4) inhibitors.

Traditional diabetes drugs have a number of disadvantages compared to incretin-based therapy. They are linked to weight loss and have been demonstrated to enhance cardiovascular outcomes in diabetic individuals. In comparison to insulin therapy, they also have a lower risk of hypoglycemia.

7. Hybrid Closed-Loop Systems, number

Algorithm-driven dosage modifications are a component of hybrid closed-loop systems, which combine CGM and insulin pump therapy. Since these devices may modify insulin delivery based on glucose readings and other factors including meal intake and physical activity, they enable more automated and individualized diabetes management.

Clinical investigations have demonstrated that hybrid closed-loop devices enhance glucose regulation and lower the chance of hypoglycemia. They are especially helpful for people who have trouble controlling their blood sugar levels or who need intense insulin therapy.

8. Technology for mobile health (mHealth)

Smartphone apps, wearable gear, and other digital tools are all examples of mobile health (mHealth) technologies that can assist patients in managing their diabetes. In order to assist patients keep on top of their diabetes treatment, these technologies can offer them real-time glucose monitoring, medication reminders, nutritional tracking, and other features.

Patients with diabetes can benefit from mHealth technology in a number of ways. It can enhance communication with healthcare professionals, assist patients in keeping track of their blood glucose levels and medication compliance, and provide patients more control over their diabetes management.

9. Machine learning and artificial intelligence

Emerging technologies like artificial intelligence (AI) and machine learning have the potential to significantly affect the management of diabetes. In order to find patterns and prescribe tailored treatments, these technologies can be used to evaluate a lot of data, including glucose measurements, medication adherence, and other health parameters.

By offering patients individualized treatment plans based on their own health data, AI and machine learning have the potential to improve glucose management outcomes. In order to prevent hypoglycemia and hyperglycemic episodes, they may also be able to detect glucose variations and notify patients to them.

10. Interventions Based on Nutrition

It has been demonstrated that nutrition-based therapies, such as low-carbohydrate and extremely low-calorie diets, enhance glucose management outcomes in some diabetic patients. These diets function by lowering blood glucose levels and enhancing insulin sensitivity.

Although nutrition-based therapies may not be suitable for all diabetic individuals, they can be a beneficial supplement to established diabetes management strategies. Patients who struggle to control their glucose levels with just medication and dietary changes may find them very helpful.

CGM, closed-loop systems, GLP-1 receptor agonists, SGLT2 inhibitors, beta cell regeneration, incretin-based therapies, hybrid closed-loop systems, mHealth technology, AI and machine learning, and nutrition-based interventions are just a few of the novel glucose management techniques that have the potential to revolutionize the treatment of diabetes. These methods give patients more individualized and efficient treatment alternatives that can help them better control their blood sugar levels and lower their chance of developing diabetes-related problems.

It's crucial to keep in mind that these cutting-edge methods are still in the early stages of development and might not be suitable for all diabetic individuals. It is crucial for individuals to consult with their medical professionals frequently to choose the diabetes treatment strategy that will work best for them.

Chapter 5

Making Use Of The Glucose Breakthrough In Everyday Life

The idea of the Glucose Breakthrough has become more well-known in recent years due to its potential to enhance health and wellbeing. The premise behind it is that people can have more energy, better cognitive function, and a lower risk of developing chronic diseases by controlling their blood sugar levels. To put the Glucose Breakthrough into practice, one must adopt lifestyle modifications that promote effective blood sugar control. This book will examine the science underlying the Glucose Breakthrough and offer helpful advice for putting it into practice in everyday life.

Understanding Blood Sugar And Glucose Regulation:

It's crucial to comprehend the fundamentals of glucose and blood sugar regulation before diving into the Glucose Breakthrough. A form of sugar called glucose can be found in a wide variety of meals, including starches like bread, pasta, and fruits. When we eat carbs, our bodies convert them to glucose, which is subsequently carried to every cell in the body by the bloodstream. By directing cells to absorb glucose from the bloodstream, the hormone insulin is crucial in controlling blood sugar levels.

Our bodies may find it difficult to control blood sugar levels if we ingest too many carbohydrates or if we develop insulin resistance. High blood sugar levels may result from this, which over time may exacerbate a number of health issues, including type 2 diabetes, cardiovascular disease, and cognitive loss.

The Discover of Glucose

The Glucose Breakthrough is a theory that seeks to promote good blood sugar control by dietary and lifestyle adjustments. People may be able to experience a variety of health advantages and lower their chance of developing chronic diseases by adhering to the Glucose Breakthrough's guiding principles.

1. Give entire, nutrient-dense foods priority:

The Glucose Breakthrough is built on a diet that gives whole, nutrient-dense foods priority. Focusing on foods high in vitamins, minerals, fibre, and other healthy nutrients will help you achieve this. Whole, nutrient-rich food examples include:

- Other veggies and leafy greens
- Berries and more sugar-free fruits
- Seeds and nuts
- Sources of high-quality protein include organic poultry, wild-caught fish, and grass-fed beef
- Wholesome fats like coconut oil, avocado, and olive oil

People can help to normalize blood sugar levels and lower the risk of insulin resistance by giving certain foods first priority.

2. Eat fewer refined and processed foods:

Processed and refined diets, as opposed to full, nutrient-dense foods, can cause unhealthful blood sugar rises. These foods frequently contain large amounts of processed carbs, added sugars, and harmful fats. Examples of foods that should be limited or avoided include:

- Sugary drinks like juice and soda
- Sweets and candies
- Baked products, including pastries, cakes, and cookies
- White pasta, processed carbs, and bread
- Fried meals and other harmful fat sources

People can lessen their chance of developing high blood sugar and insulin resistance by limiting certain items.

3. Develop a mindful eating habit.

Mindful eating entails observing hunger and fullness signs as well as being focused and present when consuming food. Individuals might lessen their risk of overeating and making unhealthful food choices by engaging in mindful eating. Below are a few recommendations for practicing mindful eating:

- Eating slowly and carefully chewing
- Observing signs of fullness and hunger
- Avoiding distractions when eating, such as television or smartphones
- Being mindful and attentive while eating

4. Exercise regularly:

By boosting insulin sensitivity and encouraging the uptake of glucose by cells, regular exercise can assist to improve blood sugar homeostasis. This suggests that those who frequently exercise may be able to better control their blood sugar levels and lower their chance of developing insulin resistance. Some forms of exercise that could be especially helpful for controlling blood sugar levels include:

- Performing aerobic exercises like cycling, swimming, or jogging
- Bodyweight exercises or weightlifting are examples of resistance training.
- Interval training at a high intensity

It's crucial to remember that people should speak with a healthcare provider before beginning a new workout regimen, especially if they have any underlying medical issues.

5. Control stress:

Prolonged stress might worsen blood sugar control by raising cortisol levels and triggering inflammation. People may be able to lower their risk of developing high blood sugar and insulin resistance by controlling their stress levels. Among the methods for reducing stress are:

- Consciousness training
- Yoga and other mild kinds of exercise
- Exercises for deep breathing
- Journaling or other expressive writing techniques
- Spending time outside or doing other stress-relieving activities

6. Get adequate sleep:

Sleep has a crucial role in maintaining overall health and wellbeing, including stable blood sugar levels. While getting enough sleep might help to increase insulin sensitivity and lower the chance of developing chronic diseases, obtaining too little sleep can lead to insulin resistance and high blood sugar. Aim for at least 7-8 hours of sleep each night, and practice good sleep hygiene by staying away from screens an hour or two before bed and by making a peaceful environment for sleeping.

Implementing The Glucose Breakthrough In Daily Life: Useful Advice

Although applying the Glucose Breakthrough's concepts to daily life can initially appear daunting, with a few helpful pointers and techniques, it can eventually become a sustainable part of your routine. Here are some helpful pointers for putting the Glucose Breakthrough into practice:

1. Make a plan:

Meal planning and preparation can help you make sure you have wholesome, nutrient-dense foods available all week. Think about making meals in advance and bringing wholesome snacks to take with you. This may lessen the urge to eat processed or foods high in sugar when you're hungry.

2. Concentrate on small, enduring changes:

Adopting the Glucose Breakthrough doesn't necessitate making significant adjustments overnight. Concentrate on implementing gradual, small-scale adjustments, such as increasing the amount of vegetables you eat at each meal or replacing sugary beverages with water or herbal tea.

3. Seek support:

Putting the Glucose Breakthrough into practice can be difficult, but getting help from friends, family, or a healthcare provider can be very beneficial. Join a support group for people interested in healthy blood sugar management, or ask a friend or family member to assist you prepare meals.

4. Exercise self-compassion:

It's critical to keep in mind that changing your way of life can take time and effort. Even if you run into obstacles or setbacks, be kind to yourself and cultivate self-compassion.

The Glucose Breakthrough is a theory that, by promoting appropriate blood sugar regulation, has the potential to enhance health and wellbeing. People can lower their risk of developing chronic diseases and gain a variety of health advantages by putting an emphasis on whole, nutrient-dense foods, reducing processed and refined foods, practicing mindful eating, exercising frequently, managing stress, and getting enough sleep. The Glucose Breakthrough may require some time and preparation, but with some useful advice and tactics, it may become a dependable part of your daily routine. Keep in mind to seek out help, concentrate on tiny, sustainable adjustments, and exercise self-compassion as you go.

Guidelines for Managing Blood Glucose Levels

Not just people with diabetes, but everyone needs to regulate their blood sugar levels. Blood glucose control, however, is essential for patients with diabetes to avoid long-term consequences from the disease. Making lifestyle adjustments, such as eating a balanced diet, exercising frequently, taking medication, and keeping track of blood glucose levels, are all part of managing blood glucose levels. We'll talk about regulating blood glucose levels in this book.

1.Regularly Check Your Blood Glucose Levels: People with diabetes must regularly check their blood glucose levels. Food, medications, and physical activity are just a few of the many things that can cause blood glucose levels to change during the day. You can evaluate how these factors affect your blood glucose levels and modify your lifestyle by routinely checking your blood glucose levels. At least once a day blood glucose testing is advised, or as directed by your healthcare physician.

2. Keep a Balanced Diet:

Controlling blood sugar levels depends on eating a balanced diet. Include nutrient-dense foods like vegetables, fruits, whole grains, lean meats, and healthy fats in your diet.. Bread, pasta, and rice are examples of foods high in carbohydrates, which can significantly affect blood glucose levels. As a result, it's crucial to keep an eye on your carbohydrate intake and select healthy sources like whole grains, fruits, and vegetables. It's also vital to stay away from processed and sugary foods because they can raise blood sugar levels.

3. Take Regular Exercise:

Regular exercise improves insulin sensitivity, which enhances the body's ability to utilise insulin, lowering blood glucose levels. By enhancing muscle glucose uptake, exercise can also lower blood glucose levels. Try to engage in at least 30 minutes of moderate-intensity activity, such as brisk walking, most days of the week.. Before beginning a new fitness regimen, speak with your healthcare professional.

4. Take Prescribed medicine:

If you have diabetes, you probably need to take medicine to help control your blood sugar levels. It is crucial to take medication exactly as directed by your doctor. Blood glucose levels can fluctuate as a result of skipping or changing doses, which can have detrimental effects on health. Before making any changes, discuss any adverse effects you may be having with your healthcare professional.

5. Control Stress:

Blood sugar levels can be significantly impacted by stress. Your body creates hormones in response to stress that may raise blood glucose levels. So controlling stress is crucial to controlling blood sugar levels. Exercise, meditation, deep breathing, and soothing pursuits like reading or listening to music are all examples of stress-management techniques.

6. Get Enough Sleep:

Sleep is essential for controlling blood sugar levels. Cortisol, a hormone that can raise blood sugar levels, can increase as a result of sleep deprivation. In order to better control blood glucose levels, try to get 7-8 hours of sleep each night.

7. Maintain Hydration:

Maintaining blood glucose levels requires drinking adequate water. Maintaining hydration is crucial since dehydration can lead to an increase in blood glucose levels. Drink 8 to 10 glasses of water a day, if possible.

8. Give up Smoking:

Smoking can raise blood sugar levels improperly. Smoking is linked to an increased risk of getting diabetes, and nicotine can raise blood glucose levels. Quitting smoking can help lower blood sugar levels and lower your risk of getting long-term consequences from diabetes.

9. Educate Yourself:

Managing blood glucose levels requires knowledge. Do your best to educate yourself on diabetes, including how it affects your body, how to control blood glucose levels, and how to avoid long-term consequences. Your Dialogue with Your Healthcare Professional:

Maintaining regular communication with your doctor is crucial for controlling your blood sugar levels. Your medical professional can work with you to develop a specific plan for controlling your blood glucose levels, modify medication dosages as necessary, and keep an eye out for any potential side effects. Keep all of your scheduled appointments with your doctor, and don't forget to let them know if your symptoms or blood sugar levels change.

10. Have a Support System:

Managing blood glucose levels can be difficult, therefore it might be helpful to have a support system. This can involve close kin, close acquaintances, or a diabetes support group. It can be simpler to control blood glucose levels and maintain motivation if you have people to talk to and share experiences with.

11. Be Ready for Emergencies:

Blood sugar levels can occasionally go dangerously high or low. It is crucial to have a plan in place in order to be ready for these emergencies. This can involve wearing a medical alert bracelet, keeping glucose tablets or a snack on hand at all times, and having an emergency action plan.

12. Use technology:

Using technology to control blood sugar levels can be beneficial. You may track your blood glucose levels, keep tabs on your food intake, and even set up devices and apps to remind you to take your prescription. Consult your healthcare physician to learn about the technological choices that might be beneficial for you.

13. Maintain a Positive Attitude:

Managing blood glucose levels can be difficult, but maintaining a positive attitude is crucial. Keep your spirits up and don't let setbacks demoralize you. Keep in mind that controlling blood sugar levels is a lifelong journey, and it's good to ask for assistance when you need it.

14. Recognize When to Get Help:

Despite dietary changes and medication, blood glucose levels occasionally may be challenging to control. Seeking medical attention from your doctor is crucial if you have persistently high or low blood sugar levels or if you are exhibiting symptoms like blurred vision, frequent urination, or excessive thirst. These can be symptoms of an illness that needs medical treatment or is more serious.

For those with diabetes in particular, controlling blood glucose levels is crucial for general health and wellbeing. You can successfully control your blood glucose levels and prevent diabetes by monitoring them frequently, eating a balanced diet, exercising frequently, taking prescribed medication, managing stress, getting enough sleep, staying hydrated, giving up smoking, educating yourself, talking with your healthcare provider, having a support system, being ready for emergencies, using technology, remaining upbeat, and knowing when to get help. Keep in mind that managing blood glucose levels is a lifelong journey, and that living a healthy and meaningful life with diabetes is feasible with the correct resources and support.

Planning Your Meals For Best Glucose Control

For those with diabetes, meal planning is crucial to sustaining good glucose control. A balanced diet, frequent exercise, and medication are all essential for maintaining appropriate blood sugar levels. Meal planning can assist diabetics in making educated decisions about their dietary intake and ensuring they are getting the right balance of carbohydrates, proteins, and fats. We will go through the significance of meal planning for the best glucose management in this book, offer some advice on how to make a healthy meal plan, and present some meal planning suggestions for those with diabetes.

Why is meal planning crucial for the best glucose management?

Keeping blood sugar levels under control is essential for those with diabetes. Uncontrolled blood sugar levels can cause major problems such heart disease, stroke, nerve damage, and kidney damage. Because meal planning enables people to regulate the quantity and kind of carbs they eat, it is crucial for blood sugar management. Glucose, which is produced when carbohydrates are broken down, is subsequently taken into the circulation. The body needs insulin to move glucose from the bloodstream into the cells, where it may be used as fuel. Diabetes patients' bodies might not create enough insulin or might not utilise it appropriately. This may cause blood sugar levels to increase.

Planning meals can help diabetics control their blood sugar levels by:

- Regulating the type and intake of carbs
- Supplying a nutritionally-balanced mixture
- Maintaining regular mealtimes and portion sizes
- Lowering the likelihood of eating too much or too little
- Enhancing general wellbeing and health

Planning A Healthy Diet

For people with diabetes, developing a nutritious diet plan is essential. A balanced diet should include a variety of carbohydrates, proteins, and fats. To prevent blood sugar spikes, carbohydrates should be ingested in moderation and spaced out throughout the day. Fats are necessary for maintaining good skin and hair as well as for absorbing some vitamins, whereas protein is crucial for constructing and repairing tissues.

In Order To Make A Healthy Meal Plan, Consider The Following Advice:

1. Consult a trained dietitian: A registered dietitian can assist people with diabetes in developing a customized food plan that takes into account their unique requirements and preferences. They can also offer advice on how to read food labels, manage portions, and use different cooking techniques.

2. Pick foods that have a low glycemic index because it indicates how rapidly a food will elevate your blood sugar levels. High glycemic index foods should be avoided or consumed sparingly. Non-starchy

veggies, whole grains, and legumes are a few examples of foods with a low glycemic index.

3. Include lean protein sources: Lean protein foods can make people feel satisfied and full, such as chicken, fish, tofu, and lentils. Tissues growth and repair necessitate the presence of a protein.

4. Pick good fats: good fats can help lower cholesterol levels and lower the risk of heart disease. Some examples of these foods include avocados, nuts, seeds, and olive oil.

5. Limit processed and sugary foods: These items should be avoided or consumed in moderation because they might cause blood sugar levels to increase.

Ideas For Meal Planning

Here are some suggestions for diabetics who are meal planning:

Breakfast:

1. Greek yoghourt with fruit and almonds freshly picked
2. Oatmeal with sliced bananas, cinnamon, and almond milk
3. Eggs on toast with spinach and scrambled

Lunch:

1. Salad of grilled chicken, tomatoes, and cucumbers with mixed greens
2. Wrapped in turkey and avocado with carrot sticks on the side.
3. A side of mixed berries, full grain crackers, and lentil soup

Dinner:

1. Quinoa, roasted asparagus, and baked salmon
2. Roasted sweet potatoes, grilled chicken, and broccoli
3. Vegetable stir-fry with brown rice and tofu

Snacks:

1. Piece of apple with almond butter
2. Sticks of carrot and hummus
3. Fried chickpeas

It is significant to remember that portion control is crucial for optimum glucose control when it comes to meal planning. To prevent increases in blood sugar levels, people with diabetes should try to eat consistent portion sizes and space out their meals throughout the day.

Advice About Dining Out

People with diabetes may find it difficult to eat out. However, it is feasible to make healthy decisions while dining out with a little forethought and preparation. Here are some recommendations for diabetics dining out:

1. Prior research on the restaurant: Before you enter the restaurant, look up the menu online. This will enable you to plan your dinner in advance and give you an idea of the possibilities available.

2. Ask for changes: Don't be scared to request changes to your food. Request grilled chicken rather than fried, or a serving of steaming vegetables in place of fries, for instance.

3. Choose carefully: Instead of fried food, go for grilled, roasted, or baked options. Pick meals that feature a lot of vegetables and lean protein.

4. Consider sharing a dish with a friend or taking half of your meal home to enjoy later if you are eating out because restaurant portions can be fairly enormous.

5. Avoid sugary beverages: Instead of sugary beverages like soda or juice, use water or unsweetened tea.

For those with diabetes, meal planning is crucial to sustaining ideal glucose control. An individual's needs and preferences should be taken into account when creating a nutritious meal plan, which should include a well-balanced combination of carbohydrates, protein, and fats. People with diabetes can control their blood sugar levels and lower their risk of problems by adhering to a healthy meal plan and making wise decisions when eating out. Before making any significant dietary or lifestyle changes, it's crucial to speak with a qualified nutritionist and a medical professional.

Incorporating Regular Exercise into Your Daily Schedule

Maintaining a healthy lifestyle requires incorporating physical activity into everyday routine. Numerous advantages of regular exercise include bettering general health, lowering the danger of chronic diseases, enhancing mood, and raising vitality. However, a lot of people struggle to find the time and inspiration to work out frequently. Luckily, there are numerous methods to add physical activity to your regular routine without making changes to your hectic schedule. The advantages of physical activity, various forms of exercise, and doable strategies to fit exercise into your daily routine are all covered in this book.

Advantages Of Exercise

There are several advantages to regular physical activity for overall health and wellbeing. Here are a few of the key advantages of consistent exercise:

1. Decreases the Chance of Chronic Illness

The chance of developing chronic conditions including diabetes, heart disease, and obesity can be lowered with regular exercise. Exercise increases insulin sensitivity, which lowers the probability of type 2 diabetes. Additionally, it lowers the risk of heart disease while enhancing cardiovascular health.

2. Enhances mood

It has been shown that engaging in physical activity can improve one's mood and reduce symptoms of anxiety and depression. Endorphins are chemicals that are released by exercise that help to lower tension and elevate mood.

3. Enhances Energy Levels

By enhancing circulation and increasing oxygen delivery to the body, exercise can aid in boosting energy levels. This could reduce fatigue and increase efficiency.

4. Enhances Rest Quality

Regular exercise will assist increase the quality of sleep, which will make it simpler to get to sleep and stay asleep. This is because a sedentary lifestyle can throw off the body's internal clock, which exercise helps to reset.

Types Of Exercises

Exercise comes in a variety of forms, each of which has advantages. These are a few of the most common forms of exercise:

1. Aerobic Activity

Any workout that speeds up respiration and the heart rate is considered aerobic. Examples include swimming, dancing, cycling, and running. Exercise that is aerobic is very beneficial for enhancing cardiovascular health and calorie burning.

2. Power Training

Weights or resistance are used during strength training to increase muscle strength and endurance. Weightlifting, resistance bands, and bodyweight exercises are a few examples. Building and maintaining muscle mass, increasing bone density, and lowering the risk of injury all depend on strength training.

3. Stretching and Flexibility

Exercises that increase flexibility and range of motion also help to prevent injuries. Examples include stretching routines, yoga, and Pilates. Exercises that increase flexibility and minimize muscle imbalances are crucial for preserving joint health.

Practical Techniques For Including Exercise in Your Daily Routine

After talking about the advantages of exercise and the many types of exercise, let's look at some realistic ways to include exercise into your daily schedule:

1. Prioritize exercise

Making exercise a priority is the first step to incorporating it into your daily schedule. Treat exercise like any other essential meeting by scheduling it in your calendar. This will make it more likely that you'll fit exercise into your schedule and follow your program.

2. Begin Small

Start out slowly and progressively increase the length and intensity of your workouts if you are new to exercising. Start with quick, easy workouts and gradually build up to longer and more intense sessions over time. This will make sure that you enjoy your workouts and assist to prevent damage.

3. Pick pastimes you enjoy

It's crucial to pick things you enjoy if you want to keep up your workout schedule. Anything from dancing to swimming to hiking might count as this. Find an enjoyable hobby to engage in, and maintaining your health will seem less like a chore and more like enjoyment.

4. Make Use of Active Transportation

Active transportation is a fantastic method to fit fitness into your regular schedule without adding extra time to it. Walking, bicycling, or running errands on foot rather than driving could be examples of this. Utilizing active transportation not only encourages physical activity but also lessens carbon emissions.

5. Take Breaks and Get Up and About

It is crucial to take pauses during the day to walk around if you have a sedentary work. This might be as easy as taking a brief office stroll or performing some stretches at your desk. The detrimental effects of prolonged sitting can be mitigated by taking breaks and moving around during the day.

6. Employ technology

You can track your physical activity and get inspiration from a variety of applications and gadgets. Fitbit and Apple Watch, among other fitness trackers, can monitor your heart rate, steps taken, and calories burned throughout the day. Numerous fitness applications are also available; these provide routines, tracking, and inspiration.

7. Involve family and friends

A fantastic method to maintain motivation and make exercise more fun is to workout with friends and family. Join your pals for a weekly workout, or take the family out for a fun activity like biking or hiking.

8. Form a Habit of Exercise

Consistency and commitment are needed if you want to incorporate fitness into your everyday routine. You can make sure that exercise becomes a regular part of your schedule by making it a habit. Set small, manageable goals to start, then gradually lengthen and intensify your workouts..

9. Make a plan.

Making a schedule in advance might help you make sure you have time to exercise and avoid making excuses. Make sure you have the right tools and time allotted for your workouts by scheduling them for the coming week. This will make it more likely that you'll incorporate exercise into your daily routine.

10. Remain Inspired

Although it can be difficult, staying motivated is crucial for keeping up a regular workout schedule. Set attainable goals, monitor your progress, and treat yourself when you meet checkpoints. Find a training partner or enroll in a fitness class to help you keep accountable and motivated.

physical activity should be a regular part of your routine if you want to maintain a healthy lifestyle. Numerous advantages of regular exercise include bettering general health, lowering the danger of chronic diseases, enhancing mood, and raising vitality. There are various methods to include exercise into your everyday routine, from taking breaks and moving around the office to employing active transportation. You can make exercise a regular part of your routine and take advantage of the many advantages that come with regular physical activity by prioritizing it, starting small, and picking activities you enjoy.

Managing Glucose Levels With The Help Of Healthcare Professionals

Keeping glucose levels under control is an essential part of diabetic therapy. Diabetes is a chronic illness that afflicts millions of people globally. High blood glucose levels brought on by either insulin resistance or inadequate insulin production characterize this metabolic condition. To prevent long-term problems such neuropathy, renal damage, and cardiovascular disease, blood sugar levels must be carefully managed. Healthcare professionals are essential to the management of glucose levels in diabetic individuals. In this book, we'll talk about managing glucose levels in conjunction with medical professionals.

Types of Healthcare Professionals Involved in the Care of Diabetics

Diabetes management calls for a multidisciplinary strategy. There are various categories of healthcare professionals involved in the treatment of diabetes, including:

1. Primary care providers (PCPs): Patients with diabetes typically contact primary care physicians (PCPs) initially. They are essential in the early detection and treatment of diabetes. PCPs are in charge of informing patients about diabetes, checking blood sugar levels, and writing prescriptions for medication.

2. Endocrinologists are experts in the identification and treatment of hormonal diseases, such as diabetes. They work with patients who have trouble maintaining their glucose levels and have received specific training in handling complicated forms of diabetes, such as type 1 diabetes.

3. Healthcare professionals that specialize in educating patients about diabetes are called diabetes educators. Patients receive education on how to control their blood sugar levels through food, exercise, and medication. They also assist patients in

acquiring the skills necessary to operate insulin delivery systems and glucose monitors.

4. Healthcare professionals that specialize in nutrition are known as registered dietitians (RDs). They assist diabetic patients with meal planning so that they can achieve their dietary requirements while controlling their blood sugar levels.

5. Pharmacists: Pharmacists are medical professionals with a focus on prescription drugs. In order to ensure that patients are aware of how to take their prescriptions properly, identify any side effects, and keep an eye out for drug interactions, they work closely with patients.

Managing Glucose Levels in Collaboration with Healthcare Professionals

Patients and healthcare professionals must work together to manage glucose levels. The following are some suggestions for coordinating glucose management with medical professionals:

1. Create a positive rapport with your healthcare providers

It's crucial to build trust with your medical team if you want to effectively control your blood sugar levels. To make sure that you and your healthcare providers are on the same page, good communication is essential. It would be beneficial if you felt at ease talking to your healthcare professionals and expressing any worries. Additionally, you ought to have faith in the fact that your medical professionals are paying attention to you and taking your worries seriously.

2. Keep scheduled appointments

Keeping up with routine doctor's visits is crucial for controlling your blood sugar levels. All of your scheduled appointments, such as those with your PCP, endocrinologist, diabetes educator, and RD, should be kept. Your healthcare professionals can check your blood glucose levels during these appointments, make any required medication adjustments, and offer education and support.

3. Watch Your Blood Glucose Levels Regularly

For effective diabetic management, daily glucose monitoring is necessary. According to your healthcare providers' instructions, you should check your blood sugar levels before night, before and after meals, and before and after physical activity. You can recognize patterns in your glucose levels with regular monitoring and change your diet, exercise routine, and medication as necessary.

4. Adhere to Your Treatment Program

It's crucial to stick to your treatment plan if you want to effectively control your blood sugar levels. Medication, dietary changes, physical activity, and self-care routines could all be part of your treatment strategy. It would be beneficial if you carried out your medical professionals' recommended course of therapy. If you are having trouble adhering to your treatment regimen, discuss possible changes with your healthcare providers.

5. Keep Moving

For good glucose level management, staying active is crucial. Exercise can enhance cardiovascular health, lower blood sugar levels, and improve insulin sensitivity. If you tried to work out for at least 30 minutes most days of the week, it would be beneficial. Prior to beginning a new fitness program, you should consult with your healthcare professionals, as they can advise you on the safest exercise intensities and activities for you.

6.Control Your Diet

In order to effectively control your glucose levels, diet management is crucial. Develop a meal plan that satisfies your nutritional requirements and aids in controlling your blood sugar levels in collaboration with your healthcare professionals. To help keep your blood sugar levels steady, your meal plan should include a variety of foods from all food categories. You should also try to eat regular meals and snacks throughout the day.

7. Take Your Prescriptions as Recommended

Effective glucose level management depends on taking your prescriptions as prescribed. If your doctor has ordered insulin, be careful to take it exactly as he or she has instructed. Additionally, you should take all other medications as prescribed and consult your doctor if you have any negative effects or have trouble maintaining your drug schedule.

8. Gain knowledge about self-care practices

You can properly manage your blood sugar levels by becoming knowledgeable about self-care activities. Self-care practices include managing stress, taking your medications as prescribed, and keeping an eye on your blood sugar levels. Together with your healthcare professionals, you should create a self-care strategy that suits your needs and aids in managing your diabetes.

9. Interact with Your Healthcare Professionals

Effective glycemic management requires open communication with your medical professionals. Any changes in your blood glucose levels, any symptoms you are having, or any problems you are having following your treatment plan should be reported to your healthcare providers. Your healthcare professionals can offer advice and assistance to help you effectively manage your diabetes.

10. Stay Current

For efficient glucose management, it's crucial to stay knowledgeable about diabetes and its treatment. You should keep abreast of the most recent studies, therapies, and self-care practices that can aid in managing your diabetes. To learn more about controlling your diabetes, consult your medical professionals, sign up for support groups, or read reliable information sources.

Benefits of Managing Glucose Levels with Healthcare Professionals

Working with medical professionals to control glucose levels has various advantages, including:

1. Better glucose management

Having improved glycemic control can be attained by working with healthcare professionals. Healthcare professionals can keep an eye on your blood sugar levels, modify your treatment plan as needed, and offer support and information to help you properly manage your diabetes.

2. Complications should be avoided

Effective glucose management can reduce your risk of developing long-term consequences from diabetes, including neuropathy, renal disease, and cardiovascular disease. Working with healthcare professionals will help you spot any issues and take care of them before they worsen.

3. Improvement in Life Quality

Your quality of life can be enhanced by correctly managing your diabetes. You can lessen the signs and problems of diabetes and have a more active and meaningful life by improving glucose control.

4. Instruction and Assistance

Working with medical professionals can give you the education and assistance you need to better manage your diabetes. Healthcare professionals can give you advice on how to regulate your blood sugar levels and avoid issues through diet, exercise, medication, and self-care practices.

Achieving good diabetes management requires controlling blood sugar levels. By offering information, support, and treatment options, healthcare providers assist individuals manage their diabetes. Patients can improve their glucose control, avoid complications, enhance their quality of life, and keep up to date on the most recent advancements in diabetes management by collaborating with healthcare professionals. If you have diabetes, be careful to build a strong rapport with your medical professionals, show up for scheduled appointments, consistently check your blood glucose levels, adhere to your treatment plan, and keep knowledgeable about diabetes management.

CHAPTER 6

The Future Of Research On Glucose

An important subject with considerable consequences for human health and wellbeing is the future of glucose research. The simple sugar molecule glucose is essential for the body's energy needs and is crucial for controlling blood sugar levels. Understanding the physiological processes through which the body creates, metabolizes, and controls glucose, as well as the part that glucose plays in the onset and course of many diseases, are the main goals of research on glucose. The future of glucose research is anticipated to be shaped by a number of significant developments, including improvements in our understanding of glucose metabolism, brand-new techniques for determining blood glucose levels, and the creation of cutting-edge therapies to treat disorders associated with glucose dysregulation.

A deeper understanding of the molecular and cellular mechanisms behind glucose metabolism is probably one of the major trends in future glucose research. The study of the enzymes, proteins, and other molecules involved in the generation, transportation, and consumption of glucose within the body by scientists is already making considerable strides in this field. For instance, scientists are examining the three-dimensional architecture of glucose transporters, which carry glucose into and out of cells, using high-resolution imaging techniques. In order to improve glucose metabolism and stop the onset of disorders like diabetes, scientists are working to understand the structural and functional characteristics of these transporters.

The creation of novel techniques for determining the body's glucose levels is another significant trend in the future of glucose research. Currently, a finger-stick blood test, which entails pricking the skin and collecting a little amount of blood for analysis, is the most popular technique for determining blood glucose levels. Although this approach is straightforward and reasonably priced, patients may find it uncomfortable and inconvenient, and it may not always yield precise readings of blood glucose levels in real time. Researchers have recently created a number of new technologies for non-invasively measuring blood sugar levels, such as implantable sensors that can measure blood sugar levels in real-time and continuous glucose monitoring devices that can be applied to the skin like a patch. In the upcoming years, these technologies are probably going to become more widely accessible, making it simpler for patients to monitor their glucose levels and manage their diabetes.

The creation of novel therapies to address disorders associated with glucose dysregulation is a third theme in the future of glucose research. One of the most prevalent and dangerous conditions associated with glucose dysregulation, diabetes affects millions of individuals worldwide. Despite the fact that a variety of medications and therapies are currently available to treat diabetes, many people still experience difficulty managing their blood sugar levels and preventing the major consequences linked to the condition. In recent years, researchers have made significant strides in creating new medications and treatments that focus on particular molecular pathways involved in glucose metabolism, such as glucagon receptor antagonists, Inhibitors of sodium-glucose cotransporter-2 (SGLT2), and glucagon-like peptide-1 (GLP-1) receptor inhibitors. In clinical studies, these medications produced encouraging outcomes, and they are anticipated to become more generally available in the upcoming years, giving patients with diabetes and other conditions linked to glucose dysregulation fresh hope.

The creation of customized medicine approaches to treating glucose dysregulation is another prominent field of glucose research that is projected to have tremendous growth in the upcoming years. The majority of diabetic medications and treatments are now recommended based on broad diagnostic categories, such as type 1 or type 2 diabetes, which may not adequately reflect the underlying molecular and cellular causes of the disease in specific patients. Doctors may be able to create more targeted and individualized medicines that are suited to the particular needs of each patient by using cutting-edge genomic and proteomic technologies to comprehend the precise molecular pathways implicated in glucose dysregulation in individual individuals. Better results for patients as well as more effective and efficient therapies for disorders linked to high blood sugar may result from this.

The application of artificial intelligence and machine learning algorithms to the analysis of sizable datasets pertaining to glucose metabolism and disease is another crucial field of glucose research that is predicted to experience tremendous advancement in the upcoming years. Scientists are accumulating enormous volumes of data on the molecular and cellular processes involved in glucose metabolism and the emergence of glucose-related disorders with the advent of high-throughput technologies like next-generation sequencing and proteomics. The work of evaluating and interpreting these datasets, however, can be challenging and calls for knowledge of bioinformatics and data science as well as advanced computer techniques. Scientists may be able to find new drug targets, create more precise diagnostic tests for diseases related to glucose, and even forecast which patients are most likely to get these diseases in the first place by analyzing these datasets using machine learning algorithms and other artificial intelligence tools.

The future of glucose research is anticipated to be influenced by a number of broader social and economic variables, including shifting demographics, healthcare regulations, and cultural attitudes toward diet and exercise, in addition to these scientific and technical trends. For instance, there will be a rising need for novel therapies for diseases linked to glucose as the world's population continues to age and the prevalence of chronic illnesses like diabetes rises. The development of more effective and affordable treatments for diabetes and other glucose-related disorders may be influenced by the pressure healthcare systems face to lower costs and improve results globally. As people and communities around the world strive to embrace healthier lives and stop the onset of chronic diseases like diabetes, cultural views regarding diet and exercise may also have an impact on the direction of glucose research in the future.

The future of glucose research is likely to be marked by a number of significant trends, such as improvements in our comprehension of glucose metabolism, new techniques for determining blood glucose levels, and the creation of novel therapeutics to treat diseases associated with glucose dysregulation. These tendencies will be influenced by a variety of developments in science and technology as well as more general social and economic considerations. The future of this discipline is promising, with the ultimate aim of glucose research being to enhance human health and wellbeing by preventing and treating disorders associated with glucose dysregulation.

New Technologies for Glucose Management and Monitoring

New glucose monitoring and management technologies are completely changing how we treat diabetes. Diabetes is a long-term metabolic illness that interferes with how our bodies use glucose or blood sugar. Complications include heart disease, kidney disease, nerve damage, blindness, and amputations are possible as a result. Therefore, it is essential to carefully monitor and manage blood glucose levels.

In the past, measuring blood glucose levels required pricking the skin and taking blood. This procedure is invasive, uncomfortable, and calls for regular monitoring, which can be difficult for many diabetics. However, new technologies are making glucose management and monitoring more practical, precise, and minimally invasive. We will talk about some of the most recent technologies for managing and monitoring glucose in this book.

1.Continuous Glucose Monitoring

Using a tiny sensor implanted beneath the skin, continuous glucose monitoring (CGM) is a technique for continually monitoring blood glucose levels during the day and night. The interstitial fluid, or fluid between cells in the body, is where the sensor measures glucose levels. People with diabetes can view their glucose levels in real-time by wirelessly transmitting the data to a monitor or smartphone app.

Compared to conventional glucose monitoring techniques, CGM offers a more complete view of blood glucose levels. In order to help people with diabetes make educated decisions about insulin dosage, nutrition, and exercise, it can identify trends and patterns in glucose levels. Additionally, the CGM notifies the user when their blood glucose levels are abnormally high or low, assisting in the prevention of hypo- and hyperglycemia.

2. FGM, or Flash Glucose Monitoring

Similar to continuous glucose monitoring (CGM), flash glucose monitoring (FGM) delivers a snapshot of glucose levels when the user scans a sensor with a reader or smartphone app. The sensor, which detects interstitial fluid glucose levels, is worn on the back of the arm.

FGM offers diabetics more flexibility than conventional glucose monitoring techniques. They are able to covertly check their glucose levels without having to take blood. FGM also offers data on glucose trends, enabling diabetics to track changes in their blood sugar levels over time.

3. Non-Invasive Blood Glucose Monitoring

An developing technology called non-invasive glucose monitoring (NIGM) seeks to do away with the necessity for invasive glucose monitoring techniques like finger-stick testing. Without the need for blood samples, NIGM measures glucose levels using a variety of technologies. Some NIGM technologies use spectroscopy or optical coherence tomography, while others use the measurement of glucose levels in saliva, tears, or perspiration.

NIGM has the potential to be less uncomfortable and more practical than current glucose monitoring techniques. The NIGM devices are not yet generally accessible for commercial usage, and their accuracy varies.

4. Systems for Artificial Pancreas

An new technology called an artificial pancreas system automates the administration of insulin based on blood glucose levels by coupling a CGM with an insulin pump. The system is made up of a tiny, on-body wearable device that houses a CGM sensor, an insulin pump, and a control algorithm. To keep blood sugar levels within a target range, the control algorithm analyzes glucose data and automatically modifies insulin dosing.

Artificial pancreas systems give diabetics more individualized and precise insulin administration, lowering their risk of hypo- and hyperglycemia. They also give users more freedom and flexibility in their daily lives because the system can change the user's insulin dosage automatically while they are sleeping or exercising.

5. Smart Insulin Pens

Traditional insulin pens can now be equipped with a digital component thanks to the development of smart insulin pens. The pens have sensors that monitor the user's insulin dosage and send information to a smartphone app. The app offers the user real-time insulin tracking as well as dose-reminder notifications. To provide more precise dosage, smart insulin pens can also calculate insulin doses depending on the user's blood glucose levels and other variables.

Smart insulin pens assist diabetics in better managing their insulin dosages, lowering the possibility of consequences from inadvertent dosing. Additionally, they give users more knowledge about their insulin dose habits, enabling them to make wise choices regarding the treatment of their diabetes.

6. Implantable technology

An developing technology called implantable devices intends to deliver continuous glucose monitoring and insulin dosing without the use of external equipment. Small sensors or pumps that are implanted under the skin and interact wirelessly with an external device or smartphone app make up implantable devices.

People with diabetes now have a more covert and practical way to manage their condition thanks to implantable gadgets. Additionally, they do away with the requirement for daily insulin injections, lowering the danger of consequences from improper dose.

Implantable technology is still in its infancy, thus it is still unclear how safe and effective they will be in the long run.

7. Intelligent Contact Lenses

A new technique known as "smart contact lenses" measures the amount of glucose in tears using a tiny sensor that is integrated into the contact lens. The information is wirelessly delivered to a smartphone app, enabling persons with diabetes to continuously monitor their blood glucose levels.

Compared to conventional glucose monitoring techniques, smart contact lenses offer a more practical and minimally invasive approach of monitoring glucose levels. They also give the user more freedom and flexibility in their daily lives because they can covertly check their glucose levels without having to take blood.

However, the long-term efficacy and safety of smart contact lenses have not yet been proved because they are still in the early stages of development.

8. Artificial intelligence and machine learning

Emerging technologies like machine learning and artificial intelligence (AI) are being employed to enhance glucose management and monitoring. People with diabetes can manage their diabetes more effectively by using machine learning algorithms to examine vast volumes of glucose data and spot patterns and trends.

Additionally, AI is being utilized to create tailored diabetes treatment strategies based on details about each patient's glucose levels, insulin dosage, diet, and activity. These individualized strategies can aid diabetics in improving glucose control and lowering their risk of problems.

The way we manage diabetes is changing as a result of new glucose monitoring and management technologies. There are a number of promising technologies that promise to make it easier, more accurate, and less invasive to monitor glucose levels and manage diabetes. These include continuous glucose monitoring, flash glucose monitoring, non-invasive glucose monitoring, artificial pancreas systems, smart insulin pens, implantable devices, smart contact lenses, and machine learning and artificial intelligence.

These technologies have many advantages, but they also have certain drawbacks. Some technologies are still in the early stages of development, and it is unknown whether they will be safe or effective in the long run. Others might be expensive or demand major lifestyle adjustments.

But as technology develops, it's probable that we'll see even more creative approaches to managing and monitoring glucose levels. People with diabetes have hope thanks to these cutting-edge technology, which give them more freedom and flexibility in daily life while also enhancing their general health and quality of life.

Promising Directions For Glucose Research

Many species, including humans, use glucose as their main source of energy. Glucose is a simple sugar. It is essential for several biological activities, such as glucose synthesis, insulin signaling, and energy metabolism. The study of glucose has advanced significantly in recent years, and exciting new approaches are emerging that may result in considerable improvements in the diagnosis and treatment of a number of disorders.

We will talk about some of the exciting areas of glucose research in this book, such as glucose sensing devices, glucose transporters, and the connection between glucose and chronic illnesses including diabetes, cancer, and Alzheimer's disease.

Sensing Technologies for Glucose

For the effective management of diabetes, a chronic metabolic illness that affects millions of individuals worldwide, accurate and dependable glucose sensing technologies are essential. Finger-stick testing and continuous glucose monitoring (CGM), which are common procedures for measuring blood glucose levels, have drawbacks that make them unsuitable for long-term glucose monitoring.

The creation of non-invasive glucose detection systems is one potential area of glucose research. These technologies measure glucose levels without the need for blood samples using a variety of methods, including infrared spectroscopy, Raman spectroscopy, and optical coherence tomography.

For instance, scientists at the University of Warwick have created a non-invasive glucose sensing device that measures glucose levels in the blood veins under the tongue using a method called hyperspectral imaging. For those with diabetes, the gadget's portability and ability to measure glucose levels in real time make it a desirable option.

The creation of implanted glucose sensors is another interesting area of glucose sensing technology. The glucose levels in the interstitial fluid may be continually monitored by these tiny, wireless sensors, which are implanted beneath the skin.

For many years, the creation of implanted glucose sensors has been a focus of research, with numerous businesses producing such devices. For instance, Senseonics has created a completely implanted CGM device that can track glucose levels continuously for up to 90 days.

Transporters Of Glucose

Proteins called glucose transporters are in charge of moving glucose across cell membranes. GLUT1, GLUT2, and GLUT4 are a few of the glucose transporter proteins, and each has a unique function in glucose metabolism.

The discovery and characterisation of new glucose transporters is one potential area of glucose research. To comprehend how glucose transporters function and how they can be specifically targeted for therapeutic effects, researchers are working to better understand their structure and function.

For instance, SLC620, a novel glucose transporter protein, was recently discovered by researchers at the University of Copenhagen to play a role in glucose uptake in the small intestine. Researchers discovered that SLC6A20 is increased in individuals with type 2 diabetes, and that blocking this transporter may enhance insulin sensitivity and glucose metabolism.

The creation of glucose transporter inhibitors is another interesting area for glucose transporter research. To treat conditions like diabetes and cancer, researchers are looking for tiny compounds that can inhibit glucose transporters.

For instance, STF-31, a small chemical inhibitor of GLUT1 discovered recently by researchers at the

University of California, San Francisco, can specifically destroy cancer cells that depend on glucose for energy. STF-31 is a viable candidate for cancer therapy because the researchers discovered that it can cause cancer cell death by obstructing glucose uptake.

Diabetes And Chronic Illnesses

Research on the connection between glucose and chronic conditions like diabetes, cancer, and Alzheimer's disease is ongoing. There is mounting evidence that many diseases develop and advance as a result of dysregulated glucose metabolism.

The creation of methods to stop or treat these illnesses by focusing on glucose metabolism is one potential area of glucose research. For instance, numerous studies have demonstrated that practices that enhance glucose metabolism, such as physical activity and dietary modifications, can lower the chance of contracting chronic illnesses including diabetes, cancer, and Alzheimer's disease.

Diabetes

A chronic metabolic condition called diabetes is characterized by elevated blood glucose levels. In contrast to type 2 diabetes, which is brought on by insulin resistance and decreased insulin secretion, type 1 diabetes is brought on by the death of insulin-producing beta cells in the pancreas.

The creation of treatments that can reinstate beta cell function or encourage beta cell regeneration is a promising area of diabetes research. Numerous strategies, including as gene therapy, cell replacement treatment, and medication development, are being investigated by researchers.

For instance, scientists at the University of California, San Francisco, recently created a gene therapy strategy that can help mice with type 1 diabetes by restoring beta cell activity. The scientists delivered a gene encoding for the GLP-1 protein, which aids in beta cell survival and insulin release, using a virus. The use of gene therapy may be a promising treatment for type 1 diabetes since it enhanced glucose metabolism and decreased blood glucose levels in mice.

Cancer

Targeting glucose metabolism has emerged as a possible technique for cancer therapy because cancer cells have a high demand for glucose. Numerous studies have demonstrated that blocking glucose uptake can kill cancer cells while protecting healthy cells.

The creation of glucose-based treatments that can target cancer cells specifically is a promising area of cancer research. Researchers are looking into a number of strategies, including glucose conjugates, glycolysis inhibitors, and glucose transporter inhibitors.

As an illustration, scientists at the University of California, San Diego, recently created a glucose compound that may transport anticancer medications to cancer cells only. The anticancer medication is bonded to a glucose molecule to create a glucose conjugate, which is selectively absorbed by cancer cells through glucose transporters. The method has demonstrated good outcomes in preclinical research and may offer a potential approach to the treatment of cancer.

Alzheimer's Condition

A neurodegenerative condition called Alzheimer's is characterized by beta-amyloid plaque and neurofibrillary tangle buildup in the brain. There is mounting evidence that the onset and course of Alzheimer's disease are influenced by dysregulated glucose metabolism.

The creation of treatments that can enhance brain glucose metabolism is a promising area for Alzheimer's disease research. Numerous strategies are being investigated by researchers, such as dietary modifications, physical activity, and pharmacological development.

In a mouse model of Alzheimer's disease, for instance, researchers from the University of Southern California have demonstrated that a ketogenic diet can enhance glucose metabolism and decrease the buildup of beta-amyloid plaques. A high-fat, low-carbohydrate diet known as the ketogenic diet causes a metabolic state termed ketosis, which has been found to enhance glucose metabolism and lessen brain inflammation.

The study of glucose has advanced significantly in recent years, and exciting new approaches are emerging that may result in considerable improvements in the diagnosis and treatment of a number of disorders. Research is currently focused on developing accurate and trustworthy glucose sensing technologies, identifying and characterizing novel glucose transporters, and creating approaches to address dysregulated glucose metabolism in chronic diseases like diabetes, cancer, and Alzheimer's disease.

The health of millions of people worldwide may be significantly improved by developments in glucose research. To completely comprehend the function of glucose in health and disease, however, as well as to develop secure and efficient medicines that target glucose metabolism, much more research is required.

The Glucose Breakthrough's Potential Effects on Public Health

Any new developments in science and medicine have the potential to significantly affect public health. Therefore, any new invention or breakthrough that can enhance the health and wellbeing of people and communities is appreciated. Understanding the possible effects of glucose advances on public health has garnered more attention recently.

The body's primary energy source is glucose. Glucose is a form of sugar. It is present in many foods, such as grains, fruits, and vegetables, and is necessary for the brain and other organs to operate properly. But too much glucose in the body can result in conditions like diabetes, obesity, and heart disease.

The ability to regulate and control glucose levels in the body, which can aid in the prevention and management of many health issues, is where the potential influence of glucose discoveries on public health resides. The following are some ways that glucose breakthroughs may affect general health:

Better Control of Diabetes

Worldwide, millions of people battle the chronic condition of diabetes. High blood glucose levels result from improper insulin production or utilization, which causes it to happen. Numerous health issues, including as nerve damage, renal illness, and visual loss, can result from this.

By offering improved instruments for monitoring and controlling blood glucose levels, glucose breakthroughs can significantly contribute to the management of diabetes. For instance, the creation of continuous glucose monitoring (CGM) devices has transformed the care of diabetes by enabling people to make educated decisions regarding their food, exercise routines, and medications by delivering real-time glucose readings.

New medications that potentially target diabetes' fundamental causes, such as insulin resistance and beta-cell malfunction, are another advance. These medications can aid in enhancing glucose regulation and lowering the danger of diabetes-related complications.

Improved Management Of Obesity

Millions of individuals around the world struggle with obesity, which is another serious health issue. It happens when there is an overabundance of body fat, which can cause a number of medical issues like diabetes, heart disease, and stroke.

By introducing novel methods for controlling obesity, glucose discoveries may have an impact on public health. For instance, the creation of novel medications that can boost metabolism and decrease hunger can aid in weight loss and general health improvement.

New surgical techniques like the gastric bypass and sleeve gastrectomy have also been developed. By shrinking the stomach and restricting the amount of food that can be consumed, these treatments can aid in weight loss.

Enhancement Of Cardiovascular Health

High blood glucose levels are frequently linked to cardiovascular disease, the largest cause of death in the world. By giving new techniques for treating cardiovascular disease, glucose discoveries can improve public health.

For instance, the creation of novel medications that can combat the underlying factors that contribute to cardiovascular disease, such as high blood pressure and high cholesterol, can help lower the risk of heart attack and stroke. New surgical techniques like angioplasty and stenting, which can help restore blood flow to the heart and lower the risk of heart attack, are another development.

Better Mental Health

By enhancing mental wellness, glucose discoveries can also have an effect on the general public. High blood glucose levels have been linked to cognitive decline and other issues with mental health, according to research.

By lowering the likelihood of these issues, advances in glucose management can contribute to an improvement in mental health. For instance, the creation of novel medications that can enhance glucose regulation and lessen brain inflammation can aid in preventing cognitive decline and enhancing general mental health.

Improved General Health And Happiness

Glucose innovations have the potential to improve general health and wellbeing in addition to the specific health issues outlined above, which can have an effect on public health. For instance, better glucose control can result in more energy, better sleep, and lower stress levels, all of which can be advantageous for both physical and mental health. Furthermore, by encouraging healthy lifestyle changes, glucose breakthroughs can have an effect on public health. For instance, real-time data from CGM devices on how various diets and activities affect blood glucose levels can inspire people to make better decisions. This can lower the chance of developing a variety of illnesses, such as diabetes, obesity, and cardiovascular disease.

Finally, through lowering healthcare expenditures, glucose advances can potentially have an effect on public health. Due to the continuing management and treatment requirements for these conditions, significant healthcare expenses are shared by diabetes, obesity, and cardiovascular disease. Glucose advances can help save healthcare expenses and increase overall healthcare efficiency by enhancing glucose management and lowering the risk of various health issues.

Challenges And Things To Think About

Although there is a chance that glucose breakthroughs will significantly affect public health, there are also a number of difficulties and factors that must be taken into account. A few of these are:

New glucose management technologies and treatments might not be accessible to everyone, which can worsen health disparities and inequality.

Cost: The cost of new glycemic management technologies and therapies may prevent some people from using them.

Side Effects: Some novel medications and therapies may cause adverse reactions that compromise general health and wellbeing.

Impacts Throughout Time: New glycemic management techniques and therapies often have unanticipated long-term impacts that are not yet fully understood.

Regulation: In order to ensure the safety and effectiveness of new glucose control methods and therapies, regulations are required. This can delay the creation and accessibility of these products and treatments.

Finally, glucose advances have the potential to improve the management and prevention of numerous health issues, such as diabetes, obesity, cardiovascular disease, and cognitive impairment. Glucose breakthroughs can encourage healthier lifestyles, lower healthcare costs, and enhance general health and wellbeing by offering novel tools and therapies for glucose management.

Access, cost, side effects, long-term consequences, and regulation are just a few of the obstacles and factors that must be taken into account. In order to ensure that new tools and therapies for managing glucose are secure, efficient, and available to everyone, it is crucial to keep funding glucose research and development. We can advance healthier, happier communities and public health by doing this.

Conclusion

The book talks about a brand-new development in glucose monitoring technology that could completely change how diabetics control their blood sugar levels. The system uses a non-invasive patch to assess sweat glucose levels using a special set of enzymes. The patch is simple to use, extremely accurate, and wearable for up to two weeks at a time. Additionally, because it is wireless, users may easily check their blood sugar levels in real-time using a smartphone or other mobile device. According to the report, this ground-breaking technology has the potential to greatly raise the standard of living for diabetics by making it simpler for patients to control their disease and prevent complications.

The book also states that the new glucose monitoring patch technology has undergone comprehensive testing to guarantee its usefulness and safety. It has been under development for a number of years. It is anticipated to get regulatory approval soon, which means people might have access to it soon. According to the paper, diabetics may experience pain, inconvenience, and time-consuming side effects from the present method of glucose monitoring, which calls for frequent blood tests and finger pricks. These invasive treatments might no longer be necessary thanks to the new patch technology, which would also give diabetics a more accurate and pleasant approach to control their blood sugar levels. The book as a whole emphasizes the potential advantages of this ground-breaking technology and implies that it may have a big influence on the lives of millions of individuals with diabetes.

Effective glucose management necessitates making a concerted effort to lower blood sugar levels. This entails putting into action doable steps that will improve health outcomes and lower the danger of consequences brought on by uncontrolled blood sugar levels.

Adopting healthy lifestyle practices, such as frequent exercise, a balanced diet, and stress reduction, is a significant technique for achieving this. Additionally, it's crucial to periodically check blood glucose levels and work closely with medical professionals to create a personalized care plan that takes into account each patient's particular needs and medical background.

Maintaining optimum health and quality of life requires taking proactive measures to improve glucose management. People can lower their chance of having diabetes-related problems and enhance their general welfare by making these steps a priority. To live a healthy and meaningful life, it is crucial to take action to improve glucose management.

Ultimately, the discovery of glucose marks a tremendous improvement in our knowledge of how the body utilizes glucose and its possible effects on human health. The study of this subject has illuminated the crucial part that glucose plays in human metabolism and revealed fresh methods for better glucose control.

The significance of consistent exercise and sustaining a healthy weight in regulating glucose levels is one important finding from this study. Physical exercise can increase insulin sensitivity and aid the body in utilizing glucose more efficiently, according to studies.

The role of nutrition in glucose regulation is another crucial factor to take into account. Blood glucose levels can be spiked by some foods, such as those heavy in refined carbohydrates and sugar, while being stabilized by other foods, such as those high in fibre and protein.

Overall, the glucose discovery has emphasized the value of adopting a holistic approach to health, which includes consistent exercise, a healthy diet, and cautious glucose level management. By implementing these techniques, people can enhance their metabolic health and lower their risk of contracting long-term illnesses like type 2 diabetes and cardiovascular disease.

Despite the fact that the glucose discovery has given us crucial new knowledge about how our bodies process glucose, there is still more to discover. New methods for controlling glucose levels and avoiding associated medical issues will probably be discovered as a result of ongoing research in this area.

The wider socioeconomic consequences of the glucose discovery should also be taken into account. Understanding how to successfully manage glucose levels is becoming more and more crucial since diabetes and other glucose-related diseases are increasing in prevalence globally. The findings of this study could have a big impact on how public health policies are developed as well as how new therapies and interventions are created.

In general, the discovery of glucose represents a tremendous advancement in our comprehension of the metabolism of glucose and its effects on health. We can better regulate glucose levels and encourage improved health outcomes for people and communities by building on this research in the future.

www.ingramcontent.com/pod-product-compliance
Lightning Source LLC
Chambersburg PA
CBHW060214260726

48658CB00005BA/2029